"Knowing your metabolic type allows you to hit the bull's-eye. *Metabolize* takes the guesswork out of choosing a diet and food supplements."

—Richard Malter, Ph.D.,
licensed nutrition counselor, clinical director,
Malter Institute for Natural Development

"In order to change, you have to create change. The first step in changing your body is to identify your body type. Ken Baum gives people the ability to direct their individual accomplishments toward their overall goal."

—Crystal Powers,
personal trainer, nutritional consultant

"If the food we eat is properly metabolized, we do better at the cellular level. We are not made alike, thus the importance of eating food, in accordance with our metabolic type."

—Clarissa Vargas,
holistic health practitioner, certified nutrition counselor,
Radiance Day Spa, Pacific Beach, California

"*Metabolize* represents a program that could very well change your life. Whether you are a student, an athlete, a homemaker, or a businessman . . . whether you are already in very good health or need to make some major improvements . . . whether you have 10 pounds or 50 to lose . . . this book can help you reach your goals and make you feel better in the process."

—Mark E. Song, M.D.

Metabolize

THE PERSONALIZED PROGRAM

FOR WEIGHT LOSS

❧

KENNETH BAUM

with Richard Trubo

A PERIGEE BOOK

A Perigee Book
Published by The Berkley Publishing Group
A division of Penguin Putnam Inc.
375 Hudson Street
New York, New York 10014

Copyright © 2000 by Kenneth Baum with Richard Trubo
Book design by Tanya Maiboroda
Cover design © 2000 Walter Harper

G. P. Putnam's Sons edition: January 2000
First Perigee edition: December 2000

Perigee ISBN: 0-399-52638-2

Published simultaneously in Canada.

The Penguin Putnam Inc. World Wide Web site address is
http://www.penguinputnam.com

The Library of Congress has catalogued the G. P. Putnam's Sons edition as follows:

Baum, Kenneth.
Metabolize! : the personalized program for weight loss / by Kenneth Baum,
with Richard Trubo.
p.   cm.
Includes index.
ISBN 0-399-14590-7
1. Weight loss.   2. Energy metabolism.   3. Phenotype.   I. Title.   II. Trubo, Richard.
RM222.2.B386   2000   99-043243 CIP
613.7—dc21

Printed in the United States of America

10   9   8   7   6   5   4   3   2   1

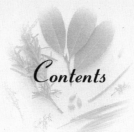

Contents

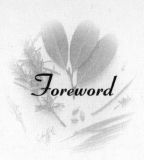

Foreword

by Mark E. Song, M.D.

Metabolize is a program that could very well change your life. Whether you are a student, an athlete, a homemaker, or a businessman . . . whether you're already in very good health or need to make some major improvements . . . whether you have 10 pounds or 50 pounds to lose . . . this book can help you reach your goals and make you feel much better in the process.

As a physician, I've always been interested in cutting-edge research that can improve people's well-being. I am chairman of the emergency department of a major medical center in Southern California, and in that capacity, I am always looking for new ways to help people who are rushed to the hospital by ambulance with their lives in the balance. At the same time, as a lifelong athlete—with 30 Ironman Triathlons to my credit—I'm also very intrigued by breakthroughs that can help ordinary people become as fit and healthy as possible. That's why I'm so impressed by the program in *Metabolize*.

I first met Ken Baum when our daughters were competing on the same volleyball team. At that time, I had already heard about Ken's work with both professional and amateur athletes and how he had been able to literally transform the careers of so many young men and women, helping them reach their full potential, no matter what their sport. I approached Ken and asked if he would meet a few times with my son, a competitive golfer who wanted to make his game even better. He agreed, and after a series of sessions, I noticed definite improvements in my son's golf game. That convinced me that Ken was doing something unique. As I became more familiar with his entire program—his emphasis on metabolic individuality, his insights into nutrition, and every other component of *Metabolize*—I began to see how his approach could help *everyone* interested in improving some aspect of his or her life.

As Ken emphasizes throughout this book, we are all unique individuals. My Metabolic Type may be different from yours. I may have different nutritional needs than you. But once you identify the lifestyle you should be leading and begin to eat, breathe, move, and think properly, you can improve your overall well-being. Very simply, this program can make you a much healthier person.

Whether you want to lose weight, increase your energy level, improve your athletic performance, or reduce your risk of serious illness now and in the future, I truly believe this book is for you. I wish you luck as you begin moving along the path toward a better and healthier life!

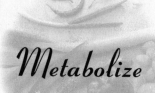

Metabolize

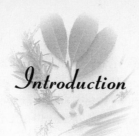

Introduction

Are you one of the millions of Americans who are obsessed with finding a way to permanently lose weight? Have you joined the pilgrimage of people in search of a proven approach for recapturing their good health? For years, I was one, too.

Even though I'd always been physically active, a flurry of unexpected and terribly painful back injuries and two major back operations limited my ability to exercise. As a result, I gained a little too much weight. Even though I never had more than 15 to 25 pounds to lose, it was always a struggle to get my waistline and the number on the bathroom scale where I wanted them. Over the years, I tried many diets, created by gurus such as Nathan Pritikin, Robert Atkins, Dean Ornish, and Barry Sears, to name a few. But nothing seemed to work for the long term. At the same time, most of my clients—from businessmen to athletes to homemakers—initially came to me to maximize their personal performance and well-being through a total mind-body approach, but they also often complained of having struggled with their weight for years. They had tried crash diets. They had fasted. They, too, hungered for a permanent solution to their health concerns.

Since the mid-1980s, I have worked with thousands of people, scanned hundreds of medical journals, and talked with dozens of researchers about cutting-edge studies in the field of weight loss and health enhancement. I went down a lot of dead ends, but in the 1990s, I came upon some of the most intriguing research I had seen. Scientists like Drs. Richard Malter, David Watts, and William Kelley had investigated various aspects of the role of metabolism in weight loss and total health and well-being. Their findings did not support what most diet gurus expound—specifically, eliminating entire categories of foods (such as carbohydrates, sugar, or meat) from the diet. Nor did their research emphasize the best way to *speed up* the body's metabolic rate on the premise that this could accelerate the burning of calories. Instead, it explored ways to improve the *overall efficiency* of metabolism by finding the ideal carbohydrate-protein-fat mix for individual metabolisms. Most intriguing, it took into account the physiological differences among individuals—that is, the biochemical characteristics that are unique to each person. This preliminary research showed that although a particular dietary plan may work for one person, it may be thoroughly inappropriate for another.

I was intrigued enough to begin collecting data of my own at my Biodynamics Institute—not only from my own clients but from thousands of people who participated in my peak-performance seminars. I also continued to compare notes with investigators like Mahlter and Watts, who were pursuing their own research at major universities and in their own treatment centers. I learned that people could be categorized into one of five Metabolic Types, which could be used to create an optimal and personalized dietary program for them. Since then, clinical experience with my own clients has shown that once their Metabolic Type is identified and they adopt the eating plan for their Type, they experience dramatic improvements in their health: They lose weight, become more energetic, improve their athletic performance, and overall feel better than they have in years.

To help them shed their excess pounds, I don't ask my clients to skip meals. Nor do they slash the number of calories they eat. They do not swallow weight-loss medications, nor exercise to the point of collapse. But in case after case, they experience improvements that persist, month after month, year after year. All they have done is determine their Metabolic Type and adjust their eating.

I tried the approach myself. I identified my Metabolic Type (I discovered that I'm a Mixed metabolizer) and then made slight adjustments to my diet. I increased my intake of protein. I modestly cut the amount of fat and carbohydrates I ate. None of these changes were hard to make. But once they were done, the efficiency of my metabolism clearly improved— and so did my health. My weight dropped from 210 to 185 pounds. At the same time, with the help of some gentle physical activity (the Seven No-Sweat Energy Movements), my back pain eased. I had more energy during the day. And I slept better at night.

The program in *Metabolize* can do the same for you. It is a breakthrough system based on principles that may be new to you but that have a strong scientific basis. In the pages that follow, you'll become acquainted with this comprehensive program and its scientific foundation. You will:

✔ Learn the principles and the science behind Metabolic Typing.

✔ Take a self-test that allows you to identify your own Metabolic Type—to determine whether you're a Super-Lean metabolizer, a Super-Clean metabolizer, or something in between.

✔ Discover the right and wrong foods for your Type, and how to adjust the ratio of dietary carbohydrates, fat, and protein in your diet to maximize your weight loss and well-being.

✔ Learn the role of vitamin and mineral supplementation in supporting your Metabolic Type.

✔ Adopt proper breathing techniques that promote metabolic efficiency and stress-busting relaxation.

✔ Use the Seven No-Sweat Energy Movements to tone, relax, stretch, and energize your body—without ever resorting to wearying exercise.

✔ Prepare your mind for success by adopting an attitude and a belief system that support dramatic improvements in your overall health.

Metabolize will help you achieve your weight-loss goals while also boosting your energy, performance, and overall good health. As you begin, make a commitment to not only read about this program but more importantly to incorporate it into your life. This book will give you the tools you need to succeed. When you make this program your own, experience it, and incorporate it into the way you eat and exercise, breathe, and think, you will enjoy the improvements that occur in your overall well-being.

Whatever your age, whatever your weight, whatever your current health status, *Metabolize* can improve the quality of your life. This is an opportunity to take responsibility for your well-being. Quite literally, your present and future health is now in your hands.

Kenneth Baum

You and Your Metabolism

Almost everyone can lose weight. In fact, most of us have done it time and time again. But within weeks or months of successfully shedding those extra five, ten, or 20 pounds, the weight invariably returns—precipitating our next attempt at losing those same excess pounds, again and again. We can lose it, but we can't keep it off.

In the same way, nearly everyone can find a way to reenergize him- or herself—at least for a while. Spend a week at a local health spa, and you'll recharge your batteries. A vacation in Hawaii or the Caribbean will do the same. But too often, after a week or a month back home in life's stressful routine, the wear and tear of everyday events takes a toll. Your stamina wanes. You feel fatigued. Burnout is back.

Then there's the issue of aging. Almost all of us have times when we feel that we're not getting older, we're getting better. But then we unexpectedly become winded after climbing a flight of stairs. Or we feel a sudden twinge of pain in our back or neck. Instantly, we're flooded with thoughts that perhaps we're losing the war against aging.

Health concerns like these can creep up on you, sometimes almost without notice. If you eat a slice of cake here, a handful of cookies there, the bathroom scale or mirror will let you know that you've overdone it. A few too many late nights at work, a daily schedule filled to overflowing with your child's car pools, soccer games, and orthodontic appointments, and you may find yourself collapsing on the couch in the evening, already dreading the stress that tomorrow will bring.

Not surprisingly, most Americans know that they aren't leading as healthy a life as they should. They acknowledge that they're not eating right. They concede that they need more exercise. "But," they rationalize, "who has the time for proper meal planning? Who has the energy for exercise?" So they look for a quick fix and enter the world of chronic dieting.

DOES ONE SIZE FIT ALL?

How many diets have you been on? If you're like most Americans, you've probably tried so many of them that D-I-E-T has become a four-letter word in your vocabulary. (It may be no coincidence that the first three letters of the word *diet* spell *die!*) But after one diet fails, there are two or three new ones to try in its place. Americans seem to have an ever-widening array of diets to choose from for managing their ever-widening waistlines. Virtually all of these eating programs have at least two things in common:

- ✔ Proponents of every new plan on the block insist that "one diet fits all"—that is, the same diet will work for everyone.
- ✔ Despite such claims, these all-purpose diets help only a small percentage of people who try them. For the rest, their chances of success are, well, slim!

No doubt about it, winning the personal battle of the bulge is a formidable challenge. We all know that. Yet each time you fail with one "miracle diet" or another, do you typically beat up on yourself? Do you tell yourself that you would have succeeded "if only I weren't such a glutton"? Or in sheer frustration, do you think, "If I just had more willpower"?

Don't be so hard on yourself. The blame actually belongs elsewhere.

This "one diet for everyone" approach is a myth, and it sets you up for failure. While the high-protein diet, the grapefruit diet, the popcorn diet, the rice diet, and every other "fad diet of the moment" may work (at least for a while) for some individuals, most people fail miserably on them. Some even *gain* weight on these programs!

It's time for a weight-loss program that acknowledges some basic facts about nutrition and our internal metabolism:

✔ Everyone has unique nutritional needs.
✔ Any single food or nutrient can have virtually an opposite biochemical effect in different people.
✔ These variations among individuals are related to differences in the way they metabolize food—that is, their *metabolic individuality*.
✔ By identifying your own unique Metabolic Type and adjusting your diet accordingly, you can avoid sabotaging your body with "one size fits all" nutrition and finally achieve your goals for weight loss and optimal health for good.

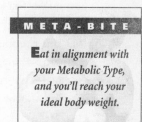

META-BITE

Eat in alignment with your Metabolic Type, and you'll reach your ideal body weight.

Chapter 2 will give you a quick course in Metabolism 101. For now, it's important to recognize that your metabolism is one of the body's most fundamental physiological processes. It determines the efficiency with which your body produces energy and burns calories. But because of metabolic uniqueness, *your* ideal diet for achieving weight loss and improvements in energy, performance, and overall health is different from the optimal diet of many other people. A particular food can have a dramatically different biochemical effect on you than on someone with a different metabolic makeup.

The idea of individual differences shouldn't be a foreign concept. All of us wear different-sized shirts, trousers, and shoes. Our physiques vary. So do our eye color, blood type, and lung capacity. Perhaps most notably, all of us have our own distinct fingerprints and dental imprints, unlike those of any other human being. So it shouldn't be surprising that one person's body's metabolism may function differently from someone else's, with characteristics that determine the efficiency with which food ultimately nourishes every cell in the body.

Your metabolism is critical in determining your overall health. You can do a lot of other health-related things right—put low-fat foods on your plate, pop vitamin pills, keep physically active, nod off for eight hours a night, purge the stress from your life—but if your diet isn't in sync with your Metabolic Type, you may still feel run-down and sickly and fight a losing battle of the bulge.

THE RISKS OF OBESITY

If weight loss is one of your health goals, you've come to the right place—and none too soon. By using the *Metabolize* program, my clients have lost the excess pounds that had stubbornly clung to them for years.

If you're obese, you are a member of a large percentage of the American population. In the early 1980s, the National Health and Nutrition Examination Survey (NHANES) found that one in four adult Americans was overweight; by the 1990s, the revised report from NHANES showed that this number had ballooned to one in three adults (about 58 million men and women!). That latest survey revealed that the average American was eight pounds plumper than he or she had been a decade earlier. That's a startling statistic, particularly in an era when more people than ever are weight-conscious and dieting and the weight-loss industry is a $2 *billion* enterprise!

Let's put the cosmetic issues aside and look at the health-related benefits of losing excess weight. If you are obese, you have an increased risk of developing one or more of the following serious chronic disorders:

- heart disease
- high blood pressure
- elevated levels of triglycerides (fats in the blood)
- certain types of cancer (of the breast, colon, rectum, uterus, ovary, prostate)
- diabetes
- gallbladder disease
- bone and joint problems (including arthritis)
- sleep apnea

Even modest weight gain can be hazardous to your health. At the Harvard School of Public Health, researchers monitored the health status of

115,000 nurses for 16 years. They found that just a moderate increase in weight—as little as 18 pounds—increased the likelihood that women would develop heart disease and cancer and have a greater risk of cardiovascular death. So if you want to stay healthy, you need to lose any extra weight you may be carrying.

Even if you're feeling healthy now, you can't count on that good fortune continuing if you're obese. Get rid of those extra pounds, however, and you'll dramatically enhance your chances of leading a long, healthy life.

METABOLISM IN ACTION

I didn't start out to help people shed their excess pounds. In the beginning, in fact, I worked primarily with world-class athletes, helping them excel in their sport through mind-body techniques and better nutrition. Very few of them were overweight. More of them looked like Jackie Joyner Kersee than Roseanne, or more like Arnold Schwarzenegger than Buddy Hackett. Yet in my interactions with them, I began to recognize that while these athletes were fit and performing at peak levels, they weren't following similar diets; in fact their diets often differed significantly. When I ate lunch with Steve Israel, the cornerback of the New England Patriots, I noticed that the primary elements of his meal were a steak and a protein drink. A few days later, when I dined with America's premier pole vaulter, Dean Starkey, he ate something quite different from Steve; his lunch included salad, chicken, vegetables, and bread. And Carl Lewis, perhaps America's greatest track star ever, concentrated on vegetarian meals!

Although they may not have been aware of it, these elite athletes were addressing their metabolic uniqueness with the food choices they made. Perhaps through trial and error, they discovered their optimal diet. But remember: What worked for one of them was probably the wrong nutritional prescription for the others. Welcome to metabolic individuality.

Here's the main point: Weight loss—as well as optimum health and longevity—are dependent on an efficiently functioning metabolism that maximizes energy production at the most basic cellular level. That, in turn, promotes proper organ and systemic activity. For optimal health, you need to respect your own Metabolic Type. Bear in mind that your Type is neither better nor worse than anyone else's. But reaching your health goals will require you to eat differently from people of other Types.

Just as our bodies are dissimilar, we shouldn't be surprised that we respond differently to various nutrients. For example, some women find that vitamin B_6 or evening primrose oil eases their PMS symptoms; for others, neither has an effect. Or at the first sneeze of winter, some individuals snuff out the sniffles with the herb echinacea or feel better taking high doses of vitamin C or plenty of grape-seed extract, while their friends have to rely solely on a box of Kleenex to get them through cold season. What works for one individual—whether it is a single nutrient or an entire diet—may undermine the health of another. So if you've failed on diets before, don't blame yourself; it was probably the wrong eating plan for your Metabolic Type.

Here's one way of thinking about this concept: You wouldn't try operating your gasoline-powered automobile on diesel fuel; in the same way, you shouldn't expect your own internal engine to run smoothly if it were being fed an inappropriate "fuel mixture" (combination of foods) for you. Unless you nurture your body with meals that are right for you, they won't be efficiently metabolized, extra calories will be stored as fat, and all of your dieting efforts, however heroic, will be in vain.

By the mid-1990s, as the *Metabolize* program crystallized, I was able to test its power in the real world. The volleyball coach at one of the University of California campuses asked me to "type" his twelve team members and analyze their diets. Everyone on the team had been eating a diet that they had chosen for themselves, based on personal preferences and habits. Sure enough, my analysis showed that, according to Metabolic Typing, only two out of the twelve should have been eating their current diet, and even those two needed to make minor adjustments. The other ten were eating so inappropriately for their Type that it was amazing that they could perform at any level.

Fortunately, all of them were willing to make adjustments in what they were eating. They simply but conscientiously followed the guidelines that you'll read about later in this book. As a result, all of the volleyball players reported feeling satisfied for longer periods after meals, without any cravings or urges to binge. They had no peaks or valleys in their energy levels. Their thinking became clearer. And those who were carrying a few extra pounds lost them.

"Can Metabolic Typing Really Help Me?"

This book presents a program that you can follow to take advantage of this new concept of Metabolic Typing. After guiding you toward determining your own unique Type, then identifying a dietary and lifestyle program based on it—with plenty of food choices to suit your personal palate and preferences—you *will* start to lose weight and improve your present and future health. That's been the experience of virtually everyone who has tried this program. It works because it addresses your biochemical individuality. At the same time, its effectiveness is maximized by paying attention to physical activity, proper breathing, and the right attitude. Rather than waiting to treat disease after it develops, it allows you to create a lifestyle for taking control of your wellness.

In my private practice, I've seen most of my clients succeed on this easy-to-follow program, using not only the optimal diet for their Type but also every other component of this well-rounded, comprehensive program. Some of these people have had serious health problems, and this plan has provided them with the optimal nutritional program that could support their healing. Others have been healthy but wanted to lose 10, 20, 30 or more pounds. So they identified their Metabolic Type. They adopted the carbohydrate-protein-fat dietary mix most appropriate for them. They integrated physical activity, proper breathing, and the right attitude into their lives. Whether they were business owners or schoolteachers, world-class athletes or homemakers, they succeeded, gradually and painlessly.

I can't repeat this often enough: A diet with a "one size fits all" philosophy won't work because it's deceiving your metabolism. It's based on the belief that we're all the same biochemically—but we're not. It claims that a single nutritional program is right for everyone—but people are different and their diets should be, too. If you've been tilting at windmills on one quick-weight-loss program after another, you've probably been downshifting your metabolism into utter chaos. Rather than getting slim fast, you may be getting fat faster. It's time for a change. Don't despair. The best diet for you *does* exist.

In Chapter 4, you'll use a self-test, a crucial element of this program, to ascertain your own Metabolic Type—whether you are a Super-Lean, Lean, Mixed, Clean, or Super-Clean metabolizer of food. Then you'll turn to easy-to-follow charts in Chapter 5 that allow you to eat according to the precisely defined ratio of carbohydrates, protein, and fat that is best for you. For some readers, the emphasis will be on carbohydrates, with a ratio of 60% carbohydrates/20% protein/20% fat; for others, their diet will put greater emphasis on protein, with an optimal ratio of 35% carbohydrates/35% protein/30% fat; still others will be eating 50% carbohydrates/25% protein/25% fat, and so on.

Let me make an important point here and perhaps ease some of your anxieties: *Metabolize* will give you plenty of food choices, despite the carefully formulated nutrient ratios. No doubt about it, eating is one of life's great pleasures. The tastes, the tactile sensations, and the colors of food all contribute to the joy of eating. If you're like me, you love to eat—you love to cook—you love the social occasions of dining with family and friends. Food is part of the celebration of being alive!

For that reason, I'm committed to balance, *not* deprivation.

With that in mind, no program can survive for long if it stresses eating primarily protein or fat, for example, at the expense of other types of food. You'll feel deprived on a diet like this, and it's not good for your metabolism. That's why this program is carefully formulated to allow every individual—no matter what his or her Metabolic Type—a large number of food choices. If you have a Super-Lean Metabolic Type, for example, you can meet your carbohydrate needs by choosing from among more than 70 vegetables and beans, over 30 fruits, and more than 50 grains.

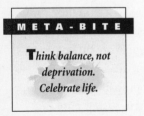

META-BITE

Think balance, not deprivation. Celebrate life.

There is a similar variety of choices for the other Metabolic Types. So if you're starting to panic about whether this is a strict, heavy-handed diet, relax. *Metabolize* is very user-friendly. It gives you many dietary choices. It calls for a regimen of physical activity that anyone can adopt. And when you eat and move this way, you will produce an internal biochemical balance and move your body in the direction of good health.

The Road to Wellville

Serious illness, whether it is associated with obesity, a poor diet, or other causes, doesn't develop overnight. It evolves gradually, perhaps over many years.

In choosing the way they live, many people aren't particularly kind to their bodies. They eat very high-fat, greasy foods . . . they're oblivious to the need for physical activity . . . they overimbibe in alcohol . . . they chain-smoke . . . they let their stress run wild. Sound familiar?

Remember, decisions you make today about your diet and your activity level can have significant health implications in the future. If you follow the *Metabolize* program for two 21-day cycles and make the choices that support good health, you can anticipate the following:

✔ A loss of *all* the excess weight that your body is carrying
✔ Renewed and sustained energy levels
✔ An easing of the physical ailments you may already have (such as back pain)
✔ Sound sleep at night
✔ Slowing the aging process and reducing the risk of developing chronic diseases such as atherosclerosis, osteoarthritis, and diabetes
✔ Better relationships and emotional balance
✔ A greater chance of a long, healthy life

You're probably thinking: "After all the diets I've tried over the years, can this one really succeed?" The answer is a resounding yes. *Metabolize* can work for you. After you've been on the program, even for just a few days, you'll begin to look and feel differently. You'll start to lose the weight you want to lose—and keep it off. And you'll feel better than you have in years.

Not long ago, a group of experts, including some at the World Health Organization, adopted the following definition of good health:

A state of well-being, of feeling good about oneself, of optimum functioning, of the absence of disease, and of the control and reduction of both internal and external risk factors for both disease and negative health conditions.

If your goal is to align your own health status with the statement above, keep in mind that you have much more control over your health than you realize. The way you feel and how long you live—and the quality of your life during those years—are, to a large degree, determined by you. *Metabolize* will help you make the right choices.

If you seize control of your well-being, you can shape your own future into a healthy one. A new way of life is awaiting you.

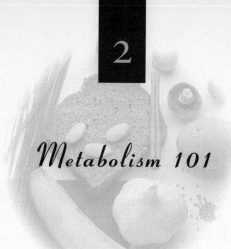

Metabolism 101

Some people check their weight every morning as routinely as they shower and brush their teeth. Their mood for the entire day is shaped by whether they've gained or lost a pound since the last time they got on the scale.

In recent years, I've worked with many clients who seem to live or die by what the scale tells them. They've often allowed all of the successes and achievements in their lives to be overshadowed by their frustration and disappointment over their "failure" to trim their weight and their waistline. They've not realized that their "failure" lay in their approach to dieting.

Until now, neither health care professionals nor the public at large have recognized the crucial role that metabolism—and specifically Metabolic Typing—can play in weight control and overall good health. People have focused solely on calories instead; biochemical individuality just hasn't been part of the picture.

In this chapter, I'll provide you with a quick course on metabolism and how it serves as the foundation of this program. But first let me introduce you to a client of mine named Marilee. She was a very successful businesswoman, running a fast-growing, thriving company. Her family relationships were strong. She had no serious health problems. By most measures, her life was very good. But she became almost inconsolable when her weight was higher than she thought it should be—which was most of the time.

For years, Marilee had struggled futilely to lose an extra thirty pounds. She had tried at least a dozen popular diets. She had gone to commercial weight-loss centers. She had spent several weeks and thousands of dollars at "fat farms" and taken virtually every known prescription and nonprescription diet pill. Time after time, her hopes rose and then were dashed. When she was on many of those diets, she felt lethargic and sluggish; on some of them, she *gained* weight. By the time she began working with me, she had just about given up. "I'm beginning to doubt that anything is ever going to work," she said.

When I recommended that we identify her Metabolic Type and that she try the eating plan customized for her, she was skeptical. It took considerable coaxing on my part. Finally, she agreed to give *Metabolize* a try, at least for a while.

We determined Marilee's Type (Lean), and then we discussed the eating plan for her. It required some adjustments to her diet. She lowered her fat intake. She raised the amount of carbohydrates she consumed. She understood that this style of eating finally gave her a real chance for successful weight loss. At the same time, she agreed to incorporate the other elements of this program—the Seven No-Sweat Energy Movements, the proper breathing techniques, and the shift in attitude—into her life.

Within a week, Marilee called with good news. Yes, she had lost three pounds—but more significantly, she said that her energy levels had increased dramatically. She sounded genuinely excited about what was happening—and that excitement actually increased during the ensuing weeks. Marilee's positive results gave her the motivation to stick with the program over the long term. She followed it for a full year (although as you'll discover, the *Metabolize* program in this book calls for a much shorter time commitment of two 21-day cycles), and she was thrilled with the results.

During that year, Marilee lost 33 pounds! At the same time as her weight loss progressed, her chronic knee pain subsided. One afternoon, as she rejoiced over her new, slimmer, healthier body, she exclaimed, "I can't believe my waistline is so skinny—and I never had to do a sit-up!"

WHAT IS METABOLISM ALL ABOUT?

When my son was quite young, I asked him, "What happens when we eat?"

Bryce's answer was succinct. "We poop!" he said.

Welcome to Metabolism 101. Bryce's explanation, of course, is not the complete story. But when I've posed the same question to dozens of adults, many knew only a little more than my son.

Actually, that's not surprising. After all, metabolism can be a complex subject. Nevertheless, I'll try to simplify it and explain how placing the proper nutrients in your body can make your metabolism more efficient and balanced.

At its most basic level, metabolism is the body's mechanism for converting nutrients into usable energy for essential everyday processes (such as rebuilding tissues and producing hormones). Food, of course, is the fuel that runs the body's engines. But a lot needs to happen to that food—including moving through all the digestive processes—before metabolism can even begin.

Of course, the steps that eventually lead to metabolism begin with that first whiff of food cooking in the oven or adorning your dinner plate. Think about the sight and smell of those delicacies and how they put your brain and body on notice that food is on its way. Just like the dog that responds to the dish placed in front of him by wagging his tail and beginning to drool, your own senses activate the salivary glands and trigger the flow of gastric juices.

When food is chewed and broken into smaller pieces, it mixes with saliva, which contains a potent enzyme (called amylase) that breaks down complex carbohydrates. Once swallowed, the food travels down the esophagus toward the stomach, avoiding an ill-advised detour into the windpipe (trachea). Through the process called peristalsis—the rhythmic contractions of the muscles of the esophagus—the food is thrust into the stomach, much as toothpaste is driven out of a tube. Once there, the stomach's powerful muscles and its chemicals shift into overdrive. The stomach's forceful churning and its relentless juices (including hydrochloric acid, the primary component of gastric juices) chemically break down the food and turn it into a partially processed, grayish semiliquid mass called chyme, which is more easily digestible. These stomach acids, by the way, are incredibly pungent and toxic; they have been compared in strength to the acids in your car's battery. But fortunately, they rarely cause injury to the stomach lining, which is well protected by layers of mucus and other protective mechanisms.

Some nutrients remain in your stomach longer than others; fats linger longer than proteins, which in turn stay longer than carbohydrates. (That's why you tend to feel satiated longer if you eat a thick slab of steak or a juicy double cheeseburger.) But gradually, in small spurts, all of the food particles (which by this point are less than one millimeter in diameter) move through a valve or gateway called the pylorus, advancing into your small intestine.

Despite its name, the small intestine isn't small at all. In fact, in most adults, it is 20 to 26 feet long! And its surface area is about the size of one-fourth of a football field! It is here, in the seemingly endless twists and turns of the small intestine, that the breakdown of food and the process of digestion finally come to a close. The intestine welcomes the chyme by bathing it in digestive juices that have arrived through ducts from the liver and pancreas. Bile, which is a fluid produced by the liver and delivered to the intestine via the gallbladder, begins to work its magic on fats, preparing them for breakdown and digestion; this process is also facilitated by digestive enzymes that are secreted by cells in the small intestine. As the chyme becomes smaller and smaller as part of the digestive process, its microscopic nutrients are absorbed into the bloodstream.

Some remaining food particles are not fully digested yet. For them, their journey is still not complete. They pass into the six-foot-long large intestine (the colon) and are finally expelled from the body as semisolid waste. Or as my son would say, "You poop!"

At last, this brings us back to the topic of metabolism. Those nutrients absorbed into the bloodstream include amino acids (broken down from proteins), fatty acids and glycerol (from fats and oils), simple sugars (from carbohydrates), and vitamins and minerals. Your bloodstream transports them to cells throughout the body. The cells are the sites where (finally!) metabolism actually takes place, producing the energy that the body needs to sustain itself and good health.

Metabolism itself is a highly complex process. Here are two of its key elements:

✔ Anabolism is the portion of metabolism in which all of the chemical changes occur that contribute to the growth and maintenance of the body. As part of this process, molecules that have made their way into cells combine with one another to form larger ones as part of the building process. Fatty acids, for example, assemble into triglycerides; amino acids join to form essential body proteins.

✔ Catabolic reactions also occur during metabolism. They have sometimes been called the "destructive" portion of metabolism. They involve the breakdown of cellular substances into simpler chemical agents that, in turn, release a high-energy compound called ATP, or adenosine triphosphate. This ATP generates heat and helps build and maintain your internal and external body.

To a large extent, whether you have an effective metabolism or one that functions less competently, it is influenced by the food choices you make. And unless those foods are supportive of your unique Metabolic Type, your metabolism is doomed to function at a suboptimal level. Remember, your body needs energy so that all of its organs and other systems work at their best. But with all the complex workings of our physiology, it's foolish to think that my body functions identically to yours, and what's best for me is best for you.

In *Metabolize*, the goal is to maximize the efficiency of your own metabolic processes—and along the way stimulate good health and minimize the storage of fat in your body. All of this requires respecting your Metabolic Type when making dietary choices.

METABOLISM'S CONTROL MECHANISMS

There are literally tens of thousands of tiny metabolic processes that occur in your body each day. Since the 1950s, however, researchers have known that despite metabolism's complexity, it falls under the control and regulation of three of the body's homeostatic systems that keep the internal physiology in balance—namely, the endocrine, autonomic and oxidative systems. Every morsel of food we eat affects us at the most basic physiological levels, sometimes stimulating our systems, other times inhibiting them. For example, most people are familiar with the influence that certain foods can have on their blood sugar level, or that sodium can have on water retention. To keep your metabolism functioning at optimal levels, and thus promoting weight loss and overall good health, your diet should maintain all of your homeostatic systems in balance. Let's look at this trio of systems more closely:

✔ **AUTONOMIC NERVOUS SYSTEM.** All physiological processes are influenced by the enormously complex nervous system. The autonomic nervous system (ANS) controls all of your body's involuntary, life-sustaining processes (breathing, heartbeat, digestion, tissue repair, immune responses), including those related to metabolism. For that reason, the ANS is crucial to your survival. It manages the heart as it pumps 2,000 gallons of blood a day, and the lungs as they breathe in 14 pints of air each minute. It affects your internal organs, glands, blood vessels, and smooth muscles—including the heart, stomach, liver, pancreas, and intestines. Overall, the nervous system contains at least 7 to 10 billion neurons (nerve cells) and is regulated by electrical impulses that travel from the brain to every part of the body.

Your autonomic nervous system has two basic operating modes: the sympathetic and the parasympathetic. The sympathetic is an energy-using system, mobilizing your body for emergencies and crises; its instinctive pattern of alarm and arousal (sometimes called the "fight or flight response") prepares you for battle against an external threat or a danger to the body. The opposing system, the parasympathetic, conserves and stores your energy and bodily resources. Its response is a condition of rest, relaxation and healing. If one of these subsets—sympathetic or parasympathetic—tends to dominate the other, it can overstimulate the ANS and throw your body chemistry, metabolism, and other bodily systems into turmoil. The ideal is a balance, which a proper diet supportive of your Metabolic Type can help maintain.

✔ **ENDOCRINE SYSTEM.** Several glands are part of this system, such as the pituitary gland in the brain, the thyroid and parathyroid glands in the neck, the adrenal glands adjacent to your kidneys, and clusters of cells (called islets of Langerhans) within the pancreas in the abdominal area, behind the stomach; the reproductive organs (ovaries, testicles) also play roles in the endocrine system. They produce and then secrete hormones directly into the bloodstream, where they are carried to every part of the body. When these hormones reach their destination—perhaps a particular organ or tissue—they attach themselves onto so-called receptors (like a key fitting into a lock) and trigger specific and life-supportive physiological activities. If the endocrine system is out of kilter, however, your metabolism and energy balance can be thrown out of sync, leaving you prone to weight gain and a variety of illnesses. Even if you restrict your calories, a weak thyroid can pack on the pounds. A malfunction of your hormone-producing glands can lead to serious illnesses, such as diabetes. Again, an optimal dietary plan can keep the endocrine system in balance.

✔ OXIDATIVE SYSTEM. The oxidative system is responsible, at the cellular level, for converting food into energy. Your own rate of oxidation reflects the efficiency with which nutrients are burned within your cells. If this oxidation rate is too slow, your metabolism will become sluggish, your food will stick around longer, and your feelings of satiation will linger. If you have an overly active oxidative system, it will disrupt your metabolism in another way; you might eat a chicken salad for dinner and feel completely satisfied—but then find yourself famished within an hour. You could end up eating five or six times a day just to satisfy your appetite.

The *Metabolize* program considers more than your oxidative style, however. The self-test in Chapter 4 will ask questions that determine your Metabolic Type by considering all the elements that influence it—your autonomic nervous system, endocrine system, oxidative system, blood type, and body type. There are plenty of elements to consider when determining your Metabolic Type. None is the entire story.

The good news is that it's not necessary to fully understand every physiological mechanism that influences whether you gain or lose weight, or feel energized or run-down. But you *do* need to recognize the crucial point that I've already made several times: There are distinctions and differences that set you apart from the people around you. Because of these differences, it may not make sense for you to eat the same foods as me. Perhaps you need to consume your nutrients in different amounts and in a unique ratio. That's why you need to identify your Metabolic Type and adopt a diet that supports the balanced functioning of all of your internal systems. The key to an efficient metabolism is eating properly—the right nutrients in the right ratios. If you consume the right fuel mixture for your Metabolic Type:

✔ Your body will become energy efficient.
✔ You will expedite weight loss.

Does Your Blood Type Make a Difference?

Blood, of course, is essential to life. It transports oxygen, nutrients, and wastes through your body. It helps maintain your body temperature at or near 98.6 degrees. It is crucial in battling infections. It facilitates the healing of wounds by forming clots.

Your blood type is one of your most distinguishing physiological characteristics. It may be A positive, for example, while people in your own family may have a different type—O, B, AB, positive or negative.

Blood type has received plenty of attention in recent years as a factor to consider when formulating your diet. According to research by James and Peter D'Adamo and other investigators, and Peter D'Adamo's book *Eat Right 4 Your Type*, blood type influences your response to particular foods. In fact, it appears that your blood type provides information on some of your optimal food choices.

When you read Chapter 4, you'll notice that the self-test determining your Metabolic Type includes a question about your blood type. Even so, the other factors that I've already discussed in this and other chapters are just as important or even more so to the overall picture and all of them are key elements to consider when determining your core Metabolic Type. Your Metabolic Type should be the primary guiding force in determining what goes on your dinner plate and what doesn't.

In Chapter 5, when you learn how to eat for your specific Metabolic Type, I'll offer some suggestions for subtle fine-tuning of your diet by considering which foods are most appropriate for people with blood types O, A, B, and AB. When you know your blood type, you can use it as one of the factors to optimize your eating plan under the *Metabolize* program.

✔ You will maximize your genetic potential for good health and longevity.

THE POWER OF METABOLIC TYPING

Metabolism and all of its complexities are key in influencing whether
you'll succeed in losing weight and optimizing your health. Now the tools
are finally available to determine whether you're consuming the best
foods (and in appropriate ratios) for your body. These food choices are
crucial for efficient metabolism. And without this kind of efficiency,
you'll encourage fat storage and become lethargic, your mental acuity will
suffer, and you may be subject to emotional highs and lows.

With the right fuel mixture, however, you can experience a real metabolic breakthrough. By eating meals with the proper ratio of protein, carbohydrates, and fat, you can maintain or restore your body's delicate
biochemical balance. As that happens, your cells will efficiently convert
calories into energy. Fewer fats will circulate in your bloodstream. You'll
create less "pollution" in your liver and other organs. In essence, your
body will have what it needs to operate at its full potential.

3

Metabolic Typing:
What Does the Science Show?

Your body was created to function in a state of good health. Wellness, in fact, is built right into every part of your physiology.

Like all people, you have developed, quite miraculously, from a single cell in your mother's uterus. And if there is a physiological intelligence within you that's smart enough to take that single cell and create a human being as complex as you are, composed of literally trillions of cells, then perhaps it's time to trust your body and fully support it with the nutrients it needs to achieve natural balance, weight control, and optimal health.

Your body has the ability to routinely heal everyday problems, such as colds, cuts, and stomachaches. Why not equip it with the nutrients it requires to maximize your capacity to stay well? No doubt about it, your physician is an important ally in your quest for good health. But *you* are your most important health provider. If you feed your body properly, it will reward you with the good health to which you're entitled.

THE POWER OF PROPER EATING

A couple years ago, I worked with a women's basketball team led by an extremely talented college coach. Her name is Sara, and she had been an all-American player during her own college years.

When Sara took charge of this college team, she knew it would be a challenge to turn a losing program around. She took a number of steps to begin that process of building a winning tradition. Sara implemented a rigorous physical training plan, aimed not only at building strength and stamina but also at perfecting the skills required for basketball. With my help, she also introduced her athletes to mental training techniques as well as proper breathing. Sure enough, the team made progress in her first year. But there was still room for more improvement.

During the off-season, all of the young women on Sara's basketball team adopted a trendy new diet that promised to enhance their performance—but their results certainly weren't uniform. Some lost weight and felt better on the plan; they had also gained some sharpness that would help them in the new season. But others fared quite differently. They actually *gained* weight on the fad diet, even though many of them had reduced the number of calories they consumed. They felt zapped of energy. They appeared to have lost an edge on the basketball court. A few even complained of having more difficulty coping emotionally with life's challenges. Not surprisingly, most of them ditched the diet. They either chose a different one, or in most cases, I convinced them to adopt *Metabolize*—with very positive results.

What happened? Why did the fad diet work for some of the athletes but not others? As I've emphasized throughout the book, the answer is simple: *One diet isn't right for everyone.* There are significant biochemical differences among people. And unless your diet is sensitive to your unique makeup, the nutrients you take in may sabotage your weight-loss goals and undermine your overall health and well-being.

Not long ago, I had been working with a group of athletes on their mental training, and I asked them to adopt the particular nutrient mix and ratio that were optimal for their Metabolic Type. They were a diverse group of men and women—a college soccer player, a university swimmer, a certified personal trainer, a professional volleyball player, and two high school athletes (in basketball and softball). Most were very serious about gaining any possible advantage in competition—and they were quite surprised when the Metabolic Type self-test showed that *none* of them had been eating in a manner that fully supported their metabolic individuality. Five of the six, in fact, needed to make a lot of modifications to reach their optimal nutrient ratios; the sixth, the personal trainer named Steve, had actually been quite close, but he still had some adjustments to make. He told me, "I've been trying to perfect my diet for almost ten years; if I had known about Metabolic Typing back then, I could have saved myself a lot of time."

EVALUATING THE RESEARCH

The notion of biochemical uniqueness has a long history, dating back to ancient Chinese and Hindu systems of medicine. Hindu tradition, for example, is rooted in acknowledging differences among individuals. Practitioners of Ayurvedic medicine, which has gained a large following in the U.S., identify three *doshas* or metabolic types, which are called *Kapha, Pitta,* and *Vata.* In her 1998 book, *The Alternative Medicine Handbook,* Barrie R. Cassileth, Ph.D., of the University of North Carolina, wrote that these *doshas* "are the bridging force among organs and internal parts of the body. . . . Although each person is believed to be a combination of characteristics from all three *doshas,* one *dosha* type predominates in each person."

According to Dr. Cassileth, the metabolic role of *doshas*

> is to keep the body intact and functional. They also maintain a balance among internal body organs. It is believed that all bodily functions are under *dosha* control. . . . Diet and therapies are prescribed on the basis of the individual's predominant *dosha* type. . . . Dietary treatments include recommendations and cautions against foods for particular *doshas.* Specific foods are thought to weaken or strengthen *doshas.*

In Western medicine, the roots of Metabolic Typing date back to the early 1900s. Francis Marion Pottenger, M.D., a University of Southern California professor and author of *Symptoms of Visceral Disease,* hypothesized that metabolic activity is controlled to a significant degree by the autonomic nervous system (which he called the vegetative or visceral nervous system). When this vegetative system is disturbed, he wrote, disease symptoms may occur. Pottenger believed that the autonomic nervous system was the underlying foundation for the metabolic uniqueness of each person. As he wrote, "The vegetative nervous system, being that system which influences those functions without which the animal cannot exist, is given an intimate and direct control over metabolic activity."

Then, beginning in the 1950s, a number of investigators explored the theory that certain food components could influence the body's key homeostatic systems—endocrine, autonomic, and oxidative. Some of the key research that, in recent years, has contributed to the formulation of *Metabolize* includes:

✔ George Watson, Ph.D., of the Lancaster Foundation for Scientific Research made the connection between oxidative processes and metabolic uniqueness. He believed that there are two "metabolic types," as he called them, that determine how "energy exchanges within the body" take place. Watson used the terms "fast oxidizer" and "slow oxidizer" to describe the way that people metabolize food. He concentrated primarily on the psychological impact of various nutritional choices, theorizing that slow and fast oxidation could produce mental and emotional reactions. In his 1972 book, *Nutrition and Your Mind,* Watson noted that "some mental illness indeed resulted from nutritional biochemical malfunctioning, since it could be entirely relieved by biochemical means." With dietary adjustments, he cited 80 percent rates of improvement in people suffering from "functional metabolic disorders." With oxidation in mind, he made recommendations of "slow-performance" and "high-performance" foods.

Watson argued that "what is optimal nutrition for one may be grossly inadequate for another." He believed that some people need to increase their intake of particular nutrients that "an ordinary 'good' diet provides. . . . Indeed, your present pattern of life may not really reflect the 'optimum you' at all, and all this can result solely from nutritional needs that you know nothing about."

But Watson recognized that just following the government's dietary allowances isn't enough, since they are based on nutritional *minimums,* not maximums. "The recommended intake of a given nutrient is usually set at about 50 percent above the bare minimum necessary for 'health,' which generally means nothing more than the absence of obvious nutritional disease," he wrote.

At the University of Texas at Austin, biochemist Roger Williams, Ph.D., reported that every human has distinct nutritional needs programmed by his or her unique genetic makeup. If these individual dietary requirements aren't met, said Williams, it can impair cellular activity and produce chronic health problems.

Williams, who also discovered one of the B vitamins (pantothenic acid) and conducted pioneering research into folic acid, created the term *biochemical individuality.* In a 1956 book by that name, he wrote,

> While the same physical mechanisms and the same metabolic processes are operating in all human bodies, the structures are sufficiently diverse and the genetically determined enzyme efficiencies vary sufficiently from individual to individual so that the sum total of all the reactions taking place in one individual's body may be very different from those taking place in the body of another individual of the same age, sex, and body size.

Based on both human and animal studies, Williams also developed what he called the "genetotrophic theory," which proposed individual nutritional requirements for people. As he pointed out, a genetotrophic condition is one that is predisposed by our genetics and triggered by nutritional factors. In his 1971 book, *Nutrition Against Disease,* he noted that a diet should not be adopted in a vacuum and that hereditary factors need to be considered. While conceding that there is still much to learn, he urged the development of methods for pinpointing each individual's unique inherited patterns, and he added, "Call it a 'metabolic profile' or any other name you wish, but plainly it represents a necessary precondition for making rational programs of nutrition tailored to fit each individual's special requirements." At the same time, he wrote, "we need . . . to establish accurate correlations between specific nutrients and the prevention of specific diseases."

According to Williams, life would be simpler if all human beings were carbon copies of one another. But, he added, "if we can apply what is known and find out more about the amounts of known and unknown nutrients that individuals need, we have in our hands marvelous tools for ushering in better health and preventing disease."

A number of other researchers have made major contributions in this field. In the mid-1970s, William D. Kelley wrote a self-published book, *The Metabolic Types.* He used some of Roger Williams's research on nutritional individuality to develop a system of typing that eventually used computer technology. Over time, it became clear that a particular control system (autonomic, oxidative, endocrine) wields more influence in each individual and strongly regulates how a particular nutrient affects a person.

Kelley is widely acknowledged as "the founder of metabolic typing as a science and a new medical paradigm," as Tom and Carole Valentine described him in their 1986 book, *Metabolic Typing: Medicine's Missing Link.* In a foreword to that book, Kelley wrote, "We would not, in our wildest nightmare, ever dream of filling the ethyl gasoline tank of our Cadillac or Rolls-Royce with diesel fuel. Yet daily we assault our bodies with the wrong nutrients. And we still expect these wonderful instruments to perform perfectly."

YOUR METABOLIC TYPE: GENETICS OR ENVIRONMENT?

Finally, after years of research, all of the pieces of the puzzle have come together into the program in this book. In the next chapter, you'll move through the steps to identify your own Metabolic Type. But is your Type really something you were born with? Or has it evolved and changed over the years?

As some of the researchers cited above believed, each person is genetically predisposed to respond to certain nutrients in particular ways. Just as you inherited so many of your characteristics—from your hair color to the hue of your skin—you were born with a Metabolic Type.

But before you rush to the phone to thank Mom and Dad for making all of this possible, here's some additional food for thought: It now appears that your core Metabolic Type *can* change. A number of factors may actually shift the way your body responds to food—creating a new Metabolic Type in which you're now operating. These Type-shifting factors include:

✔ the constant stress of everyday life
✔ pollutants (that is, toxic levels of lead or mercury, or industrial wastes)
✔ medications (including cancer chemotherapy)
✔ repeated consumption of the same food items
✔ food allergies
✔ nicotine, caffeine, and other stimulants
✔ substance abuse
✔ chronic diseases

But even though your current Metabolic Type may not be the one you were born with, it is the one that determines the way your body now responds to the foods you eat. When you take the self-test in Chapter 4, it will identify your Type, regardless of whether it was the one you inherited. (I also recommend retaking the test periodically, especially if any of the factors listed above have become part of your life.)

No matter what your Metabolic Type turns out to be, *Metabolize* will guide you toward making the food choices that are optimal for you. Walk through a supermarket, read a menu at your favorite restaurant, or drive along a highway jammed with McDonald's and Burger Kings, and you know that the food choices and the temptations around you are almost endless. You're not in an environment like that of the traditional Eskimos, for example, living in an isolated culture, eating the same high-protein, high-fat, whale-blubber-rich diet that your parents, grandparents, and many generations before them thrived on. (One Eskimo elder, in response to a question on what he liked about being alive, said, "If I were dead, I couldn't eat!") It is a far different eating style from what you would have if you were the descendant of the people native to Hunza in the northern tip of Pakistan who survived on a nonmeat diet—fruits, vegetables, grains, and nuts—for countless generations, through adaptation that began many centuries ago. But if you are more the product of the ethnic pluralism of America and our rather complicated heritages, your Metabolic Type may be less predictable and may not even be the same one that your siblings were born with. I know something about this firsthand; my two children, Brittany and Bryce, have different Types, and thus they need to eat diets with unique nutrient ratios—which makes for some interesting times in the kitchen and at the dinner table. Bryce and my wife, Barbara, can seemingly eat anything they want and never gain weight; but Brittany and I need to stick to our Metabolic Type plan to maintain our optimal body weight. In a case like this, you and your family members should be eating differently to optimize weight loss and enhance your overall health. Sure, you and your siblings could survive eating the same diet (you probably grew up with the same food on the dinner table); but maximizing your well-being may require something different.

By becoming overly dependent on modern medicine, many people have tended to deny the influence they can have on their own well-being. But you need to be willing to take control of your health destiny. The *Metabolize* diet can become a powerful pathway to good health and a more fulfilling life. By adopting the dietary program in harmony with your Metabolic Type, with the appropriate ratio of nutrients, you will burn calories far more efficiently, you will maximize your potential for ideal body weight, and you'll live longer and healthier.

4

What Is Your Metabolic Type?

Not long ago, I began working with an insurance agent named Janice. In her mid-thirties, she was about twenty pounds overweight and was a classic "stress eater"—responding to the anxiety and the pressures of her workday by eating for comfort, always on the run.

Janice's stress seemed to override all of her best intentions to stick to a low-calorie diet. She often grabbed a candy bar or a bag of potato chips just to get herself through the next appointment. Several times a year, she would latch onto the "fad diet of the moment." But invariably, when she wouldn't see quick results or would become distracted by the hectic pace of her life, she felt like a failure. "I've come to a point where I've just about resigned myself to being overweight forever," she told me with exasperation in her voice.

When Janice and I began working together, I taught her a technique to help manage her stress. She learned the Power of Breath, which calmed her nerves and allowed her to focus on what she was eating (see Chapter 8). She also took the self-test that appears later in this chapter—a questionnaire to identify her Metabolic Type. Then, with this information in hand, we began to tackle her weight problem head-on. We created an eating program—simple but specific—concentrating on foods that would provide her with an appropriate ratio of carbohydrate, protein, and fat for her Type. We also talked about the importance of sticking with the plan for 21 days. She made a commitment to the program, even blocking out time for meals in her datebook, as though she were scheduling work-related appointments.

When I checked with Janice about four weeks later, the excitement in her voice was at lottery-winning levels. She had gone beyond her initial 21-day commitment to the program and was still using it after a full month. "Why would I quit now?" she said. "I've done so well, and I've still got another ten pounds to go."

Janice admitted that she had to make some adjustments in what she ate. Because her Metabolic Type was Mixed, her dietary plan called for putting much less emphasis on some of her favorite foods, including oranges, corn, and ham. (We'll go into more detail about the diets for each Type in Chapter 5.) But she still had plenty of foods to choose from, ranging from beef to cheese to apples.

"Yes, I've had to make some changes in what I eat," Janice told me. "But once I understood the diet and got used to planning my meals each day, it quickly became a very comfortable part of my life." When we spoke most recently, Janice had reached and maintained her goal of twenty pounds lost, and she was managing the stress in her life much more successfully.

PUTTING YOUR METABOLIC TYPE TO THE TEST

By now, of course, you know how important it is to identify your Type and then to eat in a way that supports it and promotes more efficient metabolism. Remember, eating according to a Type other than your own may cause you to *gain* weight, not lose it, and to *deplete* your energy, not boost it.

If you're eating the "old-fashioned" way, you're approaching your diet as though you were randomly shooting darts with your eyes covered. Sometimes you'll hit the target, just by chance consuming those foods that are best for you. But most of the time you won't. If you switch to an eating plan in sync with your Metabolic Type, however, it's like taking off the blindfold, concentrating intently on your target, and hitting the bull's-eye *every time*.

So what's the easiest way to determine your Metabolic Type? At first glance, finding your Type might seem overly complex, simply because your internal physiological workings are much more intricate than even the most elaborate Rube Goldberg contraption. You can't guess your Type; that would be a futile process. But there *is* a way to calculate which of the major Metabolic Types is yours, and it involves taking a self-test. You might wonder how this test, which asks many questions about your dietary and lifestyle habits and preferences, as well as how your body responds to food, could determine crucial factors such as the operations of your autonomic nervous system for example, and your oxidative and endocrine systems. But take heart: The self-test is based on my research at the Biodynamics Institute. It incorporates data from evaluations of many men and women, and from scrutinizing how the body responds to various foods; it even examines personality characteristics. With a careful examination of countless case studies, and the help of sophisticated computer analysis, the questionnaire has been fine-tuned. It takes into account five elements— your oxidative, endocrine, and autonomic nervous systems, and your body type and blood type. It has been tested on people like you and has been shown to be an accurate, proven way of determining Metabolic Type.

PUTTING YOUR METABOLISM TO THE TEST

✔ In each horizontal row, put a checkmark in the box next to the most appropriate of the five descriptions.

✔ Choose only one answer (the best one) for each row.

✔ If no description in a particular category fits you, do not place a check in that row. But if an answer comes close—that is, seems to fit an inclination you have—then check that box.

✔ If you sense occasional repetition in this self-test, you're right! It is there intentionally, for confirmatory reasons. The self-test's scoring system takes this into account.

Add up the number of checkmarks in each column in this self-test, and place the cumulative totals from all the pages on the last line on

	1	2	3	4	5
Red meat makes me feel . . .	☐ Weighted down and tired	☐ Slightly heavy, losing energy	☐ Good, content	☑ Great, energized	☐ The best! Look out, world!
I gain weight . . .	☐ In a pot belly or all over equally	☐ In the thighs or rear end	☐ In the belly or upper legs	☑ In the upper body (stomach, back, rib cage)	☐ In an extreme way in the upper body
My appetite at scheduled meal-times is . . .	☐ Low and under control; I could wait an hour before eating, and remain content; I sometimes forget to eat	☐ Light; I can sense it's time to eat, but I could still wait an hour without any problem	☐ Average; I sometimes feel hungry; I may eat just because it's time, or I might choose to wait an hour	☐ Strong; I must eat; waiting an hour would be difficult and may leave me irritable and with low energy	☐ Very strong; I'm starving, irritable, and have no energy; I could eat a horse. Wait an hour? Not on your life!
I eat fruit as a snack . . .	☐ More than once a day	☐ Once daily	☐ Occasionally	☐ Rarely	☐ Almost never
Eating chicken or turkey . . .	☐ Leaves me feeling good, even if I consume just a little of it	☐ Satisfies and energizes me	☐ Leaves me feeling content; I like it	☑ Gives me energy but only when I eat a lot of it	☐ Is okay—but I'd rather have steak!
An hour after eating pasta for lunch, I feel . . .	☐ *Extremely* energized	☐ Energized and feeling good	☑ A little tired	☐ Quite sleepy	☐ Sound asleep
My personality is . . .	☐ *Extremely* curious, witty, and sociable	☑ Curious, witty, and sociable	☐ Extroverted, a real talker, the life of the party	☐ Controlling and demanding	☐ *Extremely* controlling and demanding
The perfect hamburger has . . .	☐ A meatless burger, loaded with vegetables	☐ A small, junior-sized patty, loaded with vegetables and sometimes with cheese	☑ An adult-sized patty with cheese on it and some vegetables	☐ An adult-sized patty with cheese on it, but I can take or leave the vegetables (depending on my mood)	☐ An adult- or super-sized patty with cheese (maybe double cheese), but almost never any vegetables (except perhaps pickles)
When I eat fish, I prefer it . . .	☐ Broiled or baked, although I could do without fish altogether	☐ Broiled or baked, but never fried	☐ Broiled, baked, or fried	☑ Fried, broiled, or baked, but I eat it only occasionally	☐ Fried—if I have to eat it at all
Totals	**Column 1 =**	**Column 2 =**	**Column 3 =**	**Column 4 =**	**Column 5 =**

	1	2	3	4	5
Eating candy or fruit for energy...	☐ Is spectacular	☐ Leaves me feeling very good	☐ Is okay	☐ Gives me a burst of energy, but then it wanes quickly	▣ Gives me a *very* rapid, *very* intense burst of energy, but then I "crash" and feel hungry
I get hunger pangs...	▣ Very rarely and that are very light	▣ That are occasional and mild	☐ Sometimes when it's my normal meal-time, and that are mild to strong	▣ That are strong; I never miss a meal	☐ That are *very* strong
When it comes to red meat...	☐ I refuse to eat it	☐ I eat it only on rare occasions, but prefer not to	☐ I eat it once or twice a week and occasionally crave it	▣ I love and crave it and eat it 4 or 5 times a week	☐ It's the best! I could eat it every day!
[Women only]: My body build is naturally...	☐ Smallish, less developed; I may even appear frail	☐ Pear-shaped, curvy, a weaker upper body	☐ Long and lanky; I often appear taller than I am; I have medium strength	▣ Strong with a solid build; I'm full-chested with broad shoulders and strong legs	☐ Extremely strong and solid, with very broad shoulders and very strong legs
My blood type is...	▣ Type A	☐ Type B	☐ Type AB	☐ Type O	
I would want to put salt on my perfect meal...	☐ Never; I prefer food's natural taste—or another seasoning	☐ Not often or only a pinch; a little salt goes a long way	▣ Sometimes	☐ Because I like salt a lot; I use it to enhance the taste	☐ I love salt. It is the best seasoning on the planet!
I eat fried chicken...	☐ Never	▣ A piece or two on rare occasions	☐ At times, and I like it	☐ Frequently	☐ It's good—and much better than baked chicken
I tend to gain weight...	☐ Not at all! I'm always very trim	☐ On the lower half of my body	▣ If I don't exercise and eat right	☐ If I don't exercise often and vigorously	☐ Easily unless I really concentrate on good nutrition
My personality is...	☐ *Extremely* calm, intellectual, idealistic	☐ Calm, intellectual, idealistic	▣ Creative, lively, quick; I'm sometimes moody, perfectionistic	☐ Assertive, orderly, decisive, task-oriented	☐ Aggressive, orderly, decisive, task-oriented
Totals	**Column 1 =**	**Column 2 =**	**Column 3 =**	**Column 4 =**	**Column 5 =**

	1	2	3	4	5
I like fast foods (on a 5-point scale) . . .	☐ 5 (can't stand them)	☐ 4	☐ 3	■ 2	☐ I (absolutely love them)
I like vegetables . . .	☐ Very much; I enjoy a wide variety, eat them at every meal and even snacks	■ A lot; I eat them daily, usually with meals, occasionally as snacks	☐ Moderately well; I often eat them with dinner or perhaps have a salad for lunch	☐ Somewhat; I enjoy some varieties, especially potatoes, carrots, or corn	☐ Not very much; I'm very picky—but I absolutely love potatoes, carrots, or corn
After eating a high-fat snack or meal, my energy level . . .	☐ Becomes very sluggish; it's too heavy	☐ Slows down, so I eat just a taste	■ Is about average	☐ Increases	☐ Becomes very high
I become angry, internally or externally (on a 5-point scale) . . .	☐ 5 (rarely, and only with a lot of provocation)	■ 4	☐ 3	☐ 2	☐ 1 (very easily)
Fasting is . . .	☐ Very easy for me to do; it makes me feel great!	☐ Slightly uncomfortable, but overall I feel good	☐ Moderately uncomfortable, but I still feel okay	■ Hard for me; I find it difficult to function while fasting	☐ *Very* hard for me; I simply can't do it
Eating fruit by itself makes me feel . . .	☐ Terrific! Look out, world!	☐ Very good and energized	☐ Pretty good; I eat fruit daily	■ Even more hungry when eating it itself	☐ Extremely hungry, so I eat it only rarely by itself
My feelings about desserts are that . . .	☐ I like them most of the time	■ I love and always have room for them	☐ I can take them or leave them; it depends on the dessert	☐ I eat them occasionally if I have room	☐ I eat them rarely; I never consciously leave room for them
At a buffet, I would choose . . .	☐ Salad, fruit, pasta, vegetables—but no meat except maybe just a taste	■ A little meat, but mostly salad, fruit, and vegetables	☐ A little of everything	☐ Primarily meat; I might eat a few vegetables but won't fill up on "rabbit food"	☐ I'm a carnivore! Give me meat, meat, and more meat (and maybe some potatoes and gravy, too)!
Totals	**Column 1 =** 1	**Column 2 =** 7	**Column 3 =** 8	**Column 4 =** 8	**Column 5 =**

5   10   6   3   2

page 38. Identify the column with the highest score, and then find your Metabolic Type below:

Column 1 = Super-Lean

Column 2 = Lean

Column 3 = Mixed

Column 4 = Clean

Column 5 = Super-Clean

In nearly every individual, one column will score higher than the others. However, if you find two columns have equal scores, then choose the one closest to the center. For example, if columns 2 and 3 are tied, choose 3 (Mixed) as your Metabolic Type. If columns 4 and 5 are tied, choose 4 (Clean) since it is closer to the middle.

MOVING TO THE NEXT LEVEL

In the next chapter, you'll see how your Type lends itself to consuming a unique blend of carbohydrates, protein, and fat. Some readers will be guided toward eating a high-carbohydrate, moderate-protein, and low-fat diet; others will adopt a high-protein, low-fat, and moderate-carbohydrate diet, and so on. It all depends on your Metabolic Type.

Let me reemphasize this point: No Metabolic Type is better than any other. Your goal is not to change your Type but rather to acknowledge and accept it and to adopt the particular nutritional plan that supports your unique biochemical characteristics. Although your Type can change, you can't transform it the way you'd alter your hairstyle or your wardrobe, nor should you want to.

You are about to embark on a new way of life. It's time to stop feeling out of control. You'll soon be eating without deprivation, enjoying a full and varied menu in harmony with your Metabolic Type. Then, once you add the other key elements of this program—including proper breathing techniques and the Seven No-Sweat Energy Movements—you will notice significant and positive changes in your body.

If you take care of your body according to the guidelines in *Metabolize*, you will finally experience the life you want.

5

Eating for Your Type

If you want a healthy, slim body, you need to design a diet with the foods that will pack an Evander Holyfield–sized wallop against all the internal mechanisms that may have sabotaged your efforts in the past. That means eating in accordance with your Metabolic Type and providing every cell of your body with its most favored foods.

Ironically, many people think of food as the enemy. To them, food poses irresistible temptations and sneaks unwelcome calories into their diet, reshaping their bodies in "unsightly" ways. But food doesn't deserve to be labeled Public Enemy Number 1. All of us need food to survive. And by choosing those foods supportive of your Type, you can make food an ally, not an "enemy," maximizing your energy production and promoting your good health.

THE NUTRIENT TROIKA: CARBOHYDRATES, PROTEIN, AND FAT

When you're creating a personalized diet for the *Metabolize* program, you'll need to focus your attention on the three food components—protein, carbohydrates, and fat—that provide energy for your body. Although many of the foods you eat contain two or even three of these essential nutrients, one of them usually predominates (as you'll see on the food lists in this chapter). Let's look at each of them more closely.

CARBOHYDRATES

Carbohydrates can be divided into two general categories: *simple carbohydrates* (such as fructose and sucrose, found in refined sugar, honey, fruits, and certain vegetables); and *complex carbohydrates* or *starch* (in vegetables, rice, cereal, bread, grains, and legumes). Gram for gram, complex carbohydrates contain the same number of calories as simple carbohydrates, and both kinds provide the body with energy; carbohydrates, in fact, are more easily metabolized into energy than proteins and fats. Simple carbohydrates are readily absorbed, while the complex variety are first broken down to simple sugars before the body makes use of them.

Complex carbohydrates tend to be much better choices for most people, because of their high-fiber and low-fat content. Although people trying to lose weight often believe that certain complex carbohydrates such as pasta and potatoes need to be avoided, that isn't necessarily true, depending on your Metabolic Type.

PROTEIN

Protein has been called "the stuff of life." It is the major building material of the body. Without it, some of our most critical physiological functions—including the growth and repair of human tissue—couldn't take place. Many parts of the body, such as the muscles, brain, and blood, are composed primarily of protein. In fact, every cell of your body has some protein in it. Protein also forms the antibodies that are the front line of our immune system.

Protein is an essential part of our diet, and because the body does not store it, we need to consume it each day. Whenever you eat protein (in foods like meat, milk, cheese, beans, and rice), you're supplying the body with the raw ingredients (called amino acids) that it requires to make its own proteins, which in turn promote muscle repair and other essential functions.

Protein plays a relatively small role in energy production; no more than about ten percent of the protein you eat is converted into energy. So if you hear a coach or anyone else recommend that you load up on protein before a strenuous game or activity, simply to give you more energy, ignore the advice, because it won't help you.

FAT

Fat, in the minds of most people, is like a terrorist, creating chaos once it enters and infiltrates the body. But consider the following: Fat in modest amounts is good for you! In fact, problems with fat occur only when you consume more than your Metabolic Type needs.

Fat is present in every cell in the body, helping to maintain cell integrity. It supports the absorption of the fat-soluble vitamins (A, D, E, and K); it helps keep your nervous system and your skin healthy; and it cushions your body's organs.

Despite its negative reputation, fat provides a readily available source of energy—about 70 percent of your energy needs! Fat also tastes good— often too good—and thus it's easy to overdo it when you're attracted by its flavor and texture. But fats also contain more calories per gram than other foods; fat is actually more than twice as calorie-dense as carbohydrates and protein. (One gram of fat contains nine calories, while one gram of carbohydrates or protein contains only four calories.) So you can eat relatively little fat and still consume plenty of calories.

Here's the painful truth: If you eat more dietary fat than your Metabolic Type eating plan calls for, it can make you fat. Also, in excess, fats can interfere with efficient metabolism. They can contribute to obesity and may even play a role in the development of certain cancers (of the colon and prostate, for example) and heart disease. For these reasons, you need to avoid overdoing the amount of fat you consume. Thus, foods like bacon, deli meats, and yogurt may be choices you should eat less of (depending on your Metabolic Type). Too much fat can also make you feel absolutely terrible; eat a chunk of cheese, for example, and you might feel unusually stuffed and uncomfortable afterward.

The riskiest fats are called *saturated* fats; they *saturate* your arteries with fatty deposits and are found primarily in animal products (such as beef, pork, ham, lamb, and veal) and many dairy items (whole milk, cheese, ice cream); they create their biggest problems when portion sizes are large—for example, choosing a twelve-ounce instead of a four-ounce steak. By contrast, the *unsaturated* fats (that is, monounsaturated and polyunsaturated fats, such as olive oil, peanut oil, and sunflower oil) actually lower your LDL ("bad") cholesterol levels. Keep in mind that for your heart health, your goal is to reduce your total and LDL cholesterol (to less than 200 and 130, respectively) and raise your HDL ("good") cholesterol (to more than 35). At the same time, your cholesterol ratio (total cholesterol divided by HDL cholesterol) should be four-to-one or lower. If you eat according to the plan for your Metabolic Type, you should reach these target levels.

The key to *Metabolize* is to promote an internal physiological balance in your body by choosing the nutrients—and consuming them in the right ratios—that directly support your own Metabolic Type, as well as weight loss and your overall good health. The ideal fuel for that goal is a unique mix of this trio of nutrients. Remember, a given food can have a completely opposite influence on your body than someone with another Metabolic Type and body chemistry. For some people, a particular item may have an activating effect; it may energize them and make them feel more alert. But in others with a different Metabolic Type, the same food can have a calming effect, leaving them feeling listless and sluggish. That's why you need to be sensitive to your Type when making dietary choices and make selections with your nutrient ratios in mind. When you eat in sync with those ratios, you'll ensure that you're converting your calories into maximum energy, maintaining internal homeostasis, and encouraging your body to function at its full potential.

META-BITE

E*at the proper "fuel mixture" for your Type, and you'll function at optimal levels.*

Take a Break from Coffee Breaks

Even before your eyes fully open in the morning, you may switch on the percolator and linger over your first cup of java. It's time to change that habit.

Caffeine is a diuretic and can cause the loss of vitamins and minerals in your urine. It also disrupts the functioning of the adrenal glands, actually making it harder for you to get started in the morning. The average American drinks two to five cups of coffee a day, from instant to designer lattes. But you're much better off doing without it altogether, allowing your body to return to a state of homeostasis.

Not only should coffee be on your personal "taboo" list, stay away from all caffeine-containing foods and beverages, including soft drinks, tea, chocolate, cocoa, and even some medications. (Certain brands of aspirin, for example, have caffeine in them.) But bear in mind that you could experience a headache if you quit caffeine cold turkey; tapering your intake over a period of seven days should reduce the likelihood of this adverse effect.

WHAT SHOULD YOU BE EATING?

Now that you know your Metabolic Type, let's get down to the specifics of the ratios in which you should eat carbohydrates, proteins, and fats, and the foods you should be eating. You need to begin eating according to the plan customized for your Metabolic Type. Here are the ratios that apply to each Type, with the percentage of calories from carbohydrates, protein, and fat.

METABOLIC TYPE	CARBOHYDRATES	PROTEIN	FAT
Super-Lean	70%	15%	15%
Lean	60%	20%	20%
Mixed	50%	25%	25%
Clean	40%	30%	30%
Super-Clean	35%	35%	30%

As you look at the food choices for each Type below, you'll see key differences among them (in addition to their unique nutrient ratios). For example:

✔ The **Lean** and **Super-Lean** Types should eat a low-fat diet that has similarities to the typical Asian diet. It is high in carbohydrates, with plenty of vegetables. When it comes to meat, these Lean and Super-Lean metabolizers fare best with "lean" varieties (like white meat), as well as light fish, healthy oils (olive, flax), nonfat or low-fat dairy products, most grains, and occasionally nuts. They don't burn high-fat meats efficiently. Women are more likely to fall into these categories than men, although people from both sexes are represented in their ranks. The parasympathetic system drives both of these Types, and the pituitary is the most active of their endocrine glands; as a component of parasympathetic activity, sedating hormones are released that slow their heart rate and the digestive and other physiological processes. These people often feel lethargic and may have type B ("laid-back") personalities.

✔ The **Clean** and **Super-Clean** Types fare better on higher-fat foods than the Lean and Super-Lean Types. To metabolize their meals efficiently, they should concentrate on beef, dark poultry, wild game, and higher fat seafood; they can eat red meat and metabolize it "cleanly." The grains they eat should be those that metabolize slowly. They should eat plenty of vegetables and fruits to keep their system functioning efficiently; in fact, most of their carbohydrates should come from veggies and fruit, with a bit less emphasis on grains. When drinking juices, they should minimize portion sizes (four-ounce glasses or less, for example). They can consume dairy products, especially yogurt, but should rely on whole or low-fat varieties. When snacking, they should mix fruits or vegetables with protein—for example, peaches with cottage cheese, and an apple with cheddar cheese. The fats they eat should be drawn from quality animal protein while generally avoiding packaged fats (potato chips). Even though these diets are composed of 30 percent fat, they shouldn't cause cholesterol levels to rise in people who are, in fact, Clean or Super-Clean metabolizers. The sympathetic system is the driving force behind these Types, and the thyroid and adrenal glands are very active. These people may crave sugar and carbohydrates, and they tend to have type A ("hard-driving") personalities.

✔ The **Mixed** Type is a mixture of the other Metabolic Types. The people in this category draw characteristics from each of the other types, and their diets fall in the middle. About half of all men fall into this type.

The food choices for your Type carefully take into account your oxidative style, the functioning of your sympathetic nervous system, and the speed at which certain foods break down and are released as glucose into the bloodstream. If you are a Clean or Super-Clean metabolizer, you need to avoid most foods with a so-called "high glycemic index"; these foods produce quick rises in blood sugar and rapid bursts of energy. Instead, your ideal foods are those that move into the bloodstream gradually and thus produce only small rises in blood sugar, giving you energy over a lengthier time. By contrast, if you're a Lean or Super-Lean metabolizer, you can eat foods with a high glycemic index that are digested rapidly and give you a quick surge of energy.

Emphasize those foods that appear in the *Preferred* column for your Type (you can consume foods from this list every day), and eat those items in the *Sometimes* and *Seldom* columns less often—two to three times a week from the *Sometimes* lists, and once or twice a month from the *Seldom* lists. (In some cases, you won't find any entries in a particular category—for example, for the Super-Lean type, there are no *Preferred* meats, but only those in the *Sometimes* and *Seldom* categories). At the same time, eat a variety of foods, choosing a cross section from your lists. In the grains sections, for instance, you may find some entries that you aren't familiar with (like barley and amaranth); they're available in most health-food stores and even in some supermarkets, so for variety, give them a try.

I will provide information on combining foods as well as menu ideas in the next chapter.

SUPER-LEAN

CARBOHYDRATES (GRAINS, FRUITS, VEGETABLES)—70%

Grains

PREFERRED amaranth, artichoke pasta, barley, buckwheat, kasha, millet, oat flour, oatmeal, oats, rice (basmati, brown, wild), rice flour, rye, 100% rye bread, rye flour, Ry-Krisp, soy flour, sprouted wheat bread

SOMETIMES bulgur wheat, corn flakes, corn muffins, couscous, cream of rice, graham flour, oat bran, oat bran muffins, puffed millet, puffed rice, quinoa, rice bran, spelt noodles, spinach noodles, white rice

SELDOM crackers, Cream of Wheat, English muffins, Familia, farina, Finn crisp, flatbread, gluten-free bread, granola, Grape-Nuts, Hi-Pro bread, multigrain bread, pancakes, pumpernickel, semolina pasta, seven-grain bread, shredded wheat, wheat bagels, wheat bread, wheat germ, wheat matzos, white flour, whole wheat bread

Fruits

PREFERRED apricots, blackberries, blueberries, cherries, figs, kiwi, lemons, limes, mangoes, papaya, pineapple, plums (dark, green, red), prunes, raisins, raspberries

SOMETIMES apples, canang melon, casaba melon, citrus, cranberries, currants (black, red), dates, elderberries, figs (dried), grapefruit, grapes (all types), guava, kumquats, loganberries, muskmelon, nectarines, oranges, peaches, pears, persimmons, pomegranates, prickly pears, strawberries, tangerines, watermelon

SELDOM bananas, cantaloupe, coconut, honeydew melon, plantains

Vegetables/Beans

PREFERRED aduke beans, adzuki beans, alfalfa sprouts, artichokes, black beans, black-eyed peas, broccoli, brussels sprouts, butter beans, carrots, celery, chickpeas (garbanzo beans), chicory, collard greens, dandelion, escarole, fava beans, garlic, green beans, kale, kohlrabi, leeks, lentils, okra, olives, parsley, parsnips, peas, pinto beans, pumpkin, red onions, romaine lettuce, soybeans, Spanish onions, spinach, Swiss chard, wax beans, white beans, yellow onions

SOMETIMES asparagus, avocado, bamboo shoots, beets, Bibb lettuce, bok choy, Boston lettuce, broad beans, cannellini beans, caraway, cauliflower, chervil, coriander, corn, cucumbers, eggplant, endive, iceberg lettuce, jicama beans, mesclun lettuce, pea pods, peppers, potatoes, radishes, snap beans, snow peas, string beans, tomatoes, yams

SELDOM kidney beans, lima beans, navy beans, red beans, tamarind beans

PROTEINS (MEAT, SEAFOOD, DAIRY)—15%

Meat

SOMETIMES Cornish hen, lean pork, white meat (turkey, chicken)

SELDOM ham, lamb, leanest beef, rabbit

Seafood

PREFERRED carp, cod, grouper, mackerel, monkfish, pickerel, rainbow trout, red snapper, salmon, sardines, sea trout, silver perch, snails, white-fish, white tuna, yellow perch

SOMETIMES mahi-mahi, ocean perch, pike, porgy, red snapper, sailfish, sea bass, shark, smelt, sturgeon, swordfish, white perch

SELDOM abalone, anchovies, barracuda, bass, beluga, bluefish, catfish, caviar, clams, conch, crab, crayfish, eel, flounder, frog, gray sole, haddock, hake, halibut, herring, lobster, mussels, octopus, oysters, scallops, shad, shrimp, sole, squid, stripel, turtle

Dairy

PREFERRED egg whites, yogurt (nonfat)

SOMETIMES cheese (nonfat), cottage cheese (nonfat), yogurt (low-fat)

SELDOM cheese (low-fat), cottage cheese (low-fat), goat cheese, goat milk, kefir, milk (nonfat)

Vegetable Protein

PREFERRED garden burger (gluten-free), Rella cheese, soy cheese, soy milk, tempeh, tofu

SOMETIMES soy "meat" products

FATS (INCLUDING OILS AND NUTS)—15%

PREFERRED flaxseed oil, olive oil, olives, peanut butter*, peanuts*, pumpkin seeds, sunflower butter, sunflower seeds, walnuts

*Avoid if allergic to peanuts.

SOMETIMES almond butter, almonds, avocado, canola, cashews, chestnuts, cod liver oil, filberts, hickory nuts, macadamia nuts, pine nuts, poppy seeds, sesame seeds, tahini butter (sesame), walnuts

SELDOM Brazil nuts, butter, pistachios

LEAN

CARBOHYDRATES (GRAINS, FRUITS, VEGETABLES)—60%

Grains

PREFERRED amaranth, artichoke pasta, barley, buckwheat, kasha, millet, oat flour, oatmeal, oats, puffed rice, rice (basmati, brown, wild), rice flour, rye, rye flour, soy flour, sprouted wheat bread

SOMETIMES bulgur wheat, corn flakes, corn muffins, couscous, cream of rice, gluten-free bread, graham flour, oat bran, oat bran muffins, puffed millet, puffed rice, quinoa, rice (basmati, brown, wild), rice bran, Ry-Krisp, spinach pasta, white rice

SELDOM crackers, Cream of Wheat, English muffins, Familia, farina, Finn crisp, flatbread, granola, Grape-Nuts, Hi-Pro bread, multigrain bread, pancakes, pumpernickel, semolina pasta, seven-grain bread, shredded wheat, wheat bagels, wheat bread, wheat germ, wheat matzos, white flour, whole wheat bread

Fruits

PREFERRED apricots, blackberries, blueberries, boysenberries, cherries, figs, kiwi, lemons, limes, pineapple, plums (dark, green, red), prunes, raisins, raspberries

SOMETIMES apples, canang melon, casaba melon, citrus, cranberries, currants (black, red), dates, elderberries, figs (dried), grapefruit, grapes (all types), guava, kumquats, loganberries, melons, muskmelon, nectarines, oranges, peaches, pears, persimmons, pomegranates, prickly pears, strawberries, tangerines, watermelon

SELDOM bananas, cantaloupe, coconut, honeydew melon, plantains

Vegetables/Beans

PREFERRED aduke beans, adzuki beans, alfalfa sprouts, artichokes, black beans, black-eyed peas, broccoli, brussels sprouts, butter beans, carrots, celery, chickpeas (garbanzo beans), chicory, collard greens, dandelion, escarole, garlic, green beans, kale, kohlrabi, leeks, lentils, okra, parsley, parsnips, peas, pinto beans, pole beans, pumpkin, red onions, romaine lettuce, soybeans, Spanish onions, spinach, Swiss chard, wax beans, white beans, yellow onions

SOMETIMES asparagus, avocado, bamboo shoots, beets, Bibb lettuce, bok choy, Boston lettuce, broad beans, cannellini beans, caraway, cauliflower, chervil, coriander, corn, cucumbers, eggplant, endive, fava beans, iceberg lettuce, jicama beans, mesclun lettuce, olives, pea pods, peppers, potatoes, radishes, snap beans, snow peas, string beans, tomatoes, yams

SELDOM kidney beans, lima beans, navy beans, red beans, tamarind beans

PROTEINS (MEAT, SEAFOOD, DAIRY)—20%

Meat

PREFERRED white meat (chicken, turkey)

SOMETIMES Cornish hen, deli meat (whole cuts, nonprocessed), lean pork, leanest beef, rabbit

SELDOM ham, hamburgers, lamb

Seafood

PREFERRED carp, cod, grouper, mackerel, monkfish, pickerel, rainbow trout, red snapper, salmon, sardines, sea trout, silver perch, snails, whitefish, white tuna, yellow perch

SOMETIMES mahi-mahi, ocean perch, pike, porgy, red snapper, sailfish, sea bass, shark, smelt, sturgeon, swordfish, white perch, white tuna

SELDOM abalone, anchovies, barracuda, bass, beluga, bluefish, catfish, caviar, clams, conch, crab, crayfish, eel, flounder, frog, gray sole, haddock, hake, halibut, herring, lobster, mussels, octopus, oysters, scallops, shad, shrimp, sole, squid, stripel, turtle

Dairy

PREFERRED cottage cheese (nonfat), egg whites, yogurt (low-fat or nonfat)

SOMETIMES cheese (low-fat), cottage cheese (low-fat), goat cheese, goat milk, kefir, milk (nonfat), whole eggs

SELDOM milk (low-fat)

Vegetable Protein

PREFERRED garden burger, soy cheese, soy "meat" products (no gluten), soy milk, tempeh, tofu

FATS (INCLUDING OILS & NUTS)—20%

PREFERRED flaxseed oil, olive oil, olives, peanut butter, peanuts, pumpkin seeds, sunflower butter, sunflower seeds, walnuts

SOMETIMES almonds, almond butter, avocado, canola, cashews, chestnuts, cod liver oil, filberts, hickory, macadamia nuts, pine nuts, poppy seeds, sesame seeds, tahini butter

SELDOM Brazil nuts, butter, pistachios

MIXED

CARBOHYDRATES (GRAINS, FRUITS, VEGETABLES)—50%

Grains

PREFERRED amaranth, barley flour, basmati rice, brown rice, brown rice bread, millet, oat bran, oat flour, oatmeal, oats, rice bran, rice flour, Ry-Krisp, 100% rye bread, rye flour, soy flour bread, sprouted wheat bread

SOMETIMES artichoke pasta, barley flour, cream of rice, granola, kamut, millet, oat-bran muffins, puffed millet, puffed rice, pumpernickel, quinoa, rice bran, rice flour, spinach pasta, Wasa bread, whole grains, wild rice

SELDOM bagels, buckwheat, bulgur wheat, corn flakes, cornmeal, corn muffins, couscous, Cream of Wheat, English muffin, Familia, farina, Finn crisp, flatbread, gluten flour, Grape-Nuts, pasta (spinach, artichoke), rice cakes, semolina pasta, seven-grain bread, shredded wheat, wheat, wheat bran, wheat bran muffins, wheat germ, wheat matzos, white flour, white rice, whole wheat bread

Fruits

PREFERRED apple, apricots, black cherries, blackberries, boysenberries, cherries, elderberries, figs, gooseberries, grapes (all types), lemons, limes, loganberries, papaya, peaches, pears, pineapple, plums, prunes, raspberries, watermelon

SOMETIMES banana, blueberries, canang melon, casaba melon, cranberries, crenshaw melon, currants (black, red), dates, figs, grapefruit, guava, honeydew melon, kiwi, kumquat, mangoes, muskmelon, nectarines, plantains, pomegranates, raisins, red dates, Spanish melon

SELDOM cantaloupe, coconut, honeydew, oranges, strawberries, tangerines

Vegetables/Beans

PREFERRED aduke beans, adzuki beans, artichokes, asparagus, black beans, black-eyed peas, broccoli, carrots, celery, chicory, collard greens, dandelion, escarole, garlic, green beans, green peas, kale, kohlrabi, leeks, okra, parsley, parsnips, pea pods, pinto beans, pole beans, pumpkin, red onions, romaine lettuce, soybeans, Spanish onions, spinach, string beans, Swiss chard, turnips, yellow onions

SOMETIMES alfalfa sprouts, arugula, avocado, bamboo shoots, beans (red, white), beets, Bibb lettuce, bok choy, Boston lettuce, broad beans, brussels sprouts, butter beans, cabbage (white, red, Chinese), cannellini beans, chervil, chickpeas, coriander, cucumbers, daikon, dill, eggplant, endive, fava beans, fennel, garbanzo beans, ginger, green onions, iceberg lettuce, jalapeños, jicama beans, kidney beans, lentils, lima beans, mesclun lettuce, mung sprouts, mushrooms (abalone, enoki, oyster, portobello, shiitake), mustard greens, navy beans, northern beans, olives, peppers (red, yellow, green), potatoes, radicchio, radishes, radish sprouts, rappini, scallions, seaweed, shallots, snap beans, snow peas, squash, sweet potatoes, tamarind seaweed, shallots, snap beans, snow peas, squash, sweet potatoes, tamarind beans, tomatoes, water chestnuts, watercress, wax beans, yams, yellow onions, zucchini

SELDOM red potatoes, white corn, white potatoes, yellow corn

PROTEINS (MEAT, SEAFOOD, DAIRY)—25%

Meat

PREFERRED beef, buffalo, chicken (dark), Cornish hen, elk, emu, lamb, mutton, ostrich, turkey (dark), venison, white meat (chicken, turkey, lean pork)

SOMETIMES duck; pheasant; pork; quail

SELDOM beef heart, kidney, liver, tongue; bacon, deli meat, ham; tripe

Seafood

PREFERRED bass (freshwater), cod, crayfish, hake, halibut, herring, mackerel, pike, rainbow trout, red snapper, salmon, sardines, sea trout, sole, sturgeon, swordfish, tilefish, tuna (dark), yellow perch

SOMETIMES anchovies, bluefish, carp, crab, crayfish, eel, flounder, frog, grouper, haddock, lobster, mahi-mahi, monkfish, ocean perch, octopus, pickerel, porgy, sailfish, scallops, sea bass, shad, shark, shrimp, silver perch, smelt, snails, squid, striped bass, tuna (light), white perch, whitefish

SELDOM abalone, barracuda, beluga, bluegill bass, catfish, caviar, clams, conch, lox, mussels, oysters, turtle

Dairy

PREFERRED cheese (low-fat, nonfat), cottage cheese (low-fat, nonfat), cream, kefir, yogurt (low-fat, nonfat)

SOMETIMES goat cheese, goat milk

SELDOM cheese (whole), milk (whole), yogurt (whole)

Vegetable Protein

PREFERRED garden burger, soy cheese, soy milk, tempeh, tofu

SOMETIMES soy "meat" products

FATS (INCLUDING OILS AND NUTS)—25%

PREFERRED almond butter, cashews, cashew butter, flaxseed oil, macadamia nuts, olive oil, pumpkin seeds, walnuts, walnut oil

SOMETIMES almonds, avocado, butter, canola oil, chestnuts, cod liver oil, filberts, hickory nuts, olives, peanut butter, peanuts, pecans, pine nuts, sesame butter, sesame seeds, sunflower butter, sunflower seeds, tahini butter

SELDOM Brazil nuts, pistachios

CLEAN

CARBOHYDRATES (GRAINS, FRUITS, VEGETABLES)—40%

Grains

PREFERRED barley, barley flour, oatmeal, quinoa, Ry-Krisp, 100% rye bread, rye flour, soy flour bread, sprouted wheat bread

SOMETIMES amaranth, artichoke pasta, basmati rice, brown rice, buckwheat, cream of rice, kamut, kasha, millet, oat bran muffins, puffed millet, puffed rice, rice bran, rice flour, spelt flour, spinach pasta, wild rice

SELDOM bagels, corn flakes, cornmeal, corn muffins, Cream of Wheat, English muffins, Familia, farina, Finn crisp, gluten-free bread, Grape-Nuts, oat bran muffins, pasta, semolina pasta, seven-grain bread, shredded wheat, wheat, wheat bran, wheat bran muffins, wheat flour, wheat germ, white rice, whole wheat bread

Fruits

PREFERRED apple, black cherries, blueberries, boysenberries, cranberries, elderberries, figs, gooseberries, grapes (red, Concord), lemons, limes, loganberries, papaya, peaches, pears, pineapple, plums, prunes, raspberries, watermelon

SOMETIMES bananas, black currants, canang melon, casaba melon, cherries, crenshaw melon, grapefruit, grapes (black, green), guava, kiwi, kumquats, mangoes, muskmelon, nectarines, persimmons, pomegranates, prickly pears, raisins, red cherries, red currants, red dates, Spanish melon, star fruit

SELDOM blackberries, cantaloupe, coconut, honeydew, oranges, rhubarb, strawberries, tangerines

Vegetables/Beans

PREFERRED aduke beans, adzuki beans, artichokes, asparagus, avocado, black-eyed peas, broccoli, celery, chicory, collard greens, dandelion, escarole, garlic, green beans, green peas, kale, kohlrabi, leeks, lentils, okra, parsley, parsnips, pea pods, pinto beans, pumpkin, red onions, red peppers, romaine lettuce, seaweed, Spanish onions, spinach, string beans, Swiss chard, tomatoes, turnips, yellow onions

SOMETIMES arugula, bamboo shoots, beans (white, red, black), beets, Bibb lettuce, bok choy, cannellini, caraway, carrots, chervil, coriander, cucumbers, daikon, dill, endive, fennel, ginger, green olives, green onions, green peppers, iceberg lettuce, jalapeños, lima beans, mesclun lettuce, mung sprouts, mushrooms (abalone, enoki, oyster, portobello), northern beans, olives, radicchio, rappini, rutabaga, scallions, shallots, snow peas, soybeans, squash, sweet potatoes, water chestnuts, watercress, yams, yellow peppers, zucchini

SELDOM alfalfa sprouts, brussels sprouts, cauliflower, Chinese cabbage, kidney beans, lentils, mushrooms (shiitake, domestic), mustard greens, navy beans, red cabbage, red potatoes, white cabbage, white corn, white potatoes, yellow corn

PROTEINS (MEAT, SEAFOOD, DAIRY)—30%

Meat

PREFERRED beef, buffalo, chicken (dark), elk, emu, lamb, mutton, ostrich, turkey (dark), venison, wild game

SOMETIMES chicken (white); Cornish hen; duck; ground beef; pheasant; pork; quail; rabbit; turkey (white)

SELDOM beef heart, kidney, liver, tongue; bacon, deli meats (whole cuts, nonprocessed); goose; ham; tripe

Seafood

PREFERRED bass, bluefish, cod, crab, crayfish, hake, halibut, herring, lobster, mackerel, pike, rainbow trout, red snapper, salmon, sardines, scallops, shrimp, sole, sturgeon, swordfish, tilefish, tuna (dark), yellow perch

SOMETIMES abalone, anchovies, beluga, carp, eel, flounder, frog, haddock, mahi-mahi, monkfish, ocean perch, pickerel, sailfish, sea bass, sea trout, silver perch, snails, squid

SELDOM barracuda, catfish, caviar, clams, conch, lox, mussels, octopus, oysters

Dairy

PREFERRED eggs, cheese (low-fat), cottage cheese (low-fat), yogurt (low-fat)

SOMETIMES goat cheese, milk (low-fat))

SELDOM cheese (whole), cottage cheese (whole), milk (whole), yogurt (whole)

Vegetable Protein

PREFERRED Garden burger (gluten-free), Rella cheese, soy cheese, soy milk, tempeh, tofu

SOMETIMES soy "meat" products

FATS (INCLUDING OILS AND NUTS)—30%

PREFERRED almonds, almond butter, butter, canola oil, cashews, cashew butter, flaxseed oil, macadamia nuts, olive oil, pumpkin seeds, walnuts, walnut oil

SOMETIMES chestnuts, cod liver oil, filberts, hickory nuts, pecans, pine nuts, sesame butter, sesame oils, sesame seeds, sunflower butter, sunflower oil, sunflower seeds

SELDOM Brazil nuts, peanut butter, peanuts, pistachios

SUPER-CLEAN

CARBOHYDRATES (GRAINS, FRUITS, VEGETABLES)—35%

Grains

PREFERRED barley, barley flour, quinoa, Ry-Krisp, 100% rye bread, rye flour, soy flour bread, sprouted wheat bread

SOMETIMES artichoke pasta, basmati rice, buckwheat, cream of rice, Finn crisp, oat bran muffins, oatmeal, puffed millet, pumpernickel, rice bran, rice flour, spelt flour, spinach pasta, wild rice

SELDOM bagels, corn flakes, cornmeal, corn muffins, corn tortillas, Cream of Wheat, English muffins, Familia, farina, Grape-Nuts, kasha, pasta, puffed rice, semolina pasta, seven-grain bread, shredded wheat, sprouted wheat, Wasa bread, wheat, wheat bran, wheat bran muffins, wheat flour, wheat germ, white rice, whole wheat bread

Fruits

PREFERRED apple, black cherries, blueberries, boysenberries, cranberries, elderberries, gooseberries, grapes (red, concord), lemons, limes, loganberries, peaches, pears, pineapple, plums, prunes, raspberries, watermelon

SOMETIMES apricots, bananas, black currants, canang melon, casaba melon, cherries, crenshaw melon, figs, grapefruit, grapes (black, green), guava, kiwi, kumquats, mangoes, muskmelon, nectarines, papayas, persimmons, pomegranates, prickly pears, raisins, red cherries, red currants, red dates, Spanish melon, star fruit

SELDOM blackberries, cantaloupe, coconut, honeydew, oranges, rhubarb, strawberries, tangerines

Vegetables/Beans

PREFERRED aduke beans, adzuki beans, artichokes, asparagus, avocado, black-eyed peas, broccoli, brown beans, butter beans, celery, chicory, collard greens, dandelion, escarole, garlic, green beans, green peas, kale, kohlrabi, leeks, lentils, okra, parsley, pea pods, pinto beans, pumpkin, red onions, red peppers, romaine lettuce, seaweed, soybeans, Spanish onions, spinach, string beans, Swiss chard, tomatoes, turnips, yellow onions

SOMETIMES arugula, bamboo shoots, beans (white, red, black), beets, Bibb lettuce, bok choy, cannellini, caraway, chervil, coriander, cucumbers, daikon, dill, endive, fennel, ginger, green olives, green onions, iceberg lettuce, jalapeños, mung sprouts, mushrooms (abalone, enoki, oyster, portobello), peppers (green, yellow), radicchio, rappini, rutabaga, scallions, shallots, snow peas, squash, sweet potatoes, water chestnuts, watercress, yams

SELDOM alfalfa sprouts, brussels sprouts, carrots, cauliflower, Chinese cabbage, fava beans, kidney beans, lentils, mushrooms (shiitake, domestic), mustard greens, navy beans, olives, parsnips, red cabbage, red potatoes, russet potatoes, white cabbage, white corn, yellow corn, zucchini

PROTEINS (MEAT, SEAFOOD, DAIRY)—35%

Meat

PREFERRED beef, buffalo, chicken (dark), elk, emu, lamb, mutton, ostrich, turkey (dark), venison

SOMETIMES Cornish hen; duck; pheasant; pork; quail; tripe

SELDOM bacon; beef heart, kidney, liver, tongue; chicken (white); deli meats; goose; ham; turkey (white)

Seafood

PREFERRED bass, bluefish, cod, crab, crayfish, hake, halibut, herring, lobster, mackerel, pike, rainbow trout, red snapper, salmon, sardines, scallops, shrimp, sole, sturgeon, swordfish, tilefish, tuna (dark), yellow perch

SOMETIMES abalone, anchovies, beluga, carp, eel, flounder, frog, haddock, mahi-mahi, monkfish, ocean perch, pickerel, sailfish, sea bass, sea trout, silver perch, snails, squid

SELDOM barracuda, catfish, caviar, clams, conch, lox, mussels, octopus, oysters

Dairy

PREFERRED eggs, cheese (low-fat), cottage cheese (low-fat), yogurt (low-fat)

SOMETIMES goat cheese, milk (low-fat)

SELDOM cheese (whole), cottage cheese (whole), milk (whole), yogurt (whole)

Vegetable Protein

PREFERRED soy milk, tempeh, tofu

SOMETIMES soy cheese

SELDOM soy "meat" products

FATS (INCLUDING OILS AND NUTS)—30%

PREFERRED almonds, almond butter, butter, cashews, cashew butter, flax-seed oil, macadamia nuts, olive oil, pumpkin seeds, walnuts, walnut oil

SOMETIMES canola oil, chestnuts, cod liver oil, filberts, hickory nuts, pecans, pine nuts, sesame butter, sesame oil, sesame seeds, sunflower butter, sunflower oil, sunflower seeds

SELDOM Brazil nuts, peanut butter, peanuts, pistachios

EATING IN SUPPORT OF YOUR BLOOD TYPE

Like your Metabolic Type, your blood type is a reflection of your internal chemistry. As previously mentioned, eating in a way that supports your Metabolic Type is a more important influence on weight loss and overall health than blood type. But researchers such as Peter J. D'Adamo (author of *Eat Right 4 Your Type*) have shown that your dietary needs may differ depending on your blood type, and his book is an excellent reference.

I strongly believe that the charts in this chapter, which recommend food choices and nutrient ratios for your own Metabolic Type, should receive most or all of your attention. By following the dietary guidelines for your Type, you can reach *all* of your health goals. But if you'd like to support your efforts further by stressing those foods that are in sync with your blood type as well, the following information will help. These foods, which are among those highly recommended for the blood type cited, also are approved foods for one or more of the five Metabolic Types.

FOR BLOOD TYPE O:

aduki beans, artichokes, broccoli, chicory, cod, collard greens, dandelion, escarole, essene bread, ezekiel bread, figs, flaxseed oil, garlic, kale, kohlrabi, leeks, mackerel, olive oil, okra, parsnips, plums, pumpkin, pumpkin seeds, rainbow trout, red snapper, romaine lettuce, salmon, sardines, Swiss chard, whitefish, yellow perch

FOR BLOOD TYPE A:

aduki beans, amaranth, apricots, artichokes, blackberries, blueberries, boysenberries, broccoli, buckwheat, cod, figs, kasha, lentils, mackerel, olive oil, peanuts, pineapple, plums, prunes, pumpkin seeds, rainbow trout, red snapper, salmon, sardines, tofu, yellow perch

FOR BLOOD TYPE B:

broccoli, cod, collard greens, cottage cheese, cranberries, essene bread, ezekiel bread, grapes (red, Concord), halibut, lamb, mackerel, olive oil, papaya, parsley, parsnip, pike, pineapple, plums, salmon, sardines, sole, sturgeon, venison, yogurt

FOR BLOOD TYPE AB:

broccoli, cod, cottage cheese, essene bread, ezekiel bread, garlic, lentils, olive oil, parsnips, rainbow trout, red snapper, salmon, sardines, sturgeon, yogurt

Now that you know what you should be eating, it's time to begin incorporating the dietary program into your life. In the next chapter, we'll start that process, including providing some sample menus to guide you in your new way of eating.

6

Strategies for Successful
Metabolic-Type Eating

You now have the basic information on what you should be eating and in what ratios. In this chapter, I'll give you some guidelines on implementing what you've learned. Most of my clients have described the ease with which they have been able to adopt the dietary plan presented in this book. After reading this chapter, I believe you'll feel the same way and will be able to confidently move forward to reach your weight-loss and other health goals.

To begin, I suggest having the charts for your Metabolic Type (from Chapter 5) at your side during this entire program. Refer to them when you're making shopping lists. Keep them nearby when you're making choices about what to eat at a given meal. After a while, you'll find that you won't have to refer to them as often; but (particularly in the first few days) review the charts frequently, and choose only those foods that are on them.

FINDING YOUR RATIOS

Until this program came along, I had tried a number of diets over the years. Many of them required an almost obsessive attention to the exact weight of every bit of food I ate. Frankly, nothing can spoil an eating plan more quickly than having to keep the kitchen scale nearby and weighing every morsel of food before it goes on your plate, meal after meal. Any diet that insists that you weigh all of your food will send most people running for cover. I'm often leading the stampede.

Let's put some good news on the table: You won't have to weigh and measure your food in order to eat in accordance with the *Metabolize* plan. Store your scale in the cupboard; you don't need it to determine whether you're eating nutrients in the proper ratio.

Perhaps, in an ideal world, you would find it useful to know what you're eating down to the last gram and the final ounce. That might help ensure that you are consuming food in a precise ratio of 40%/30%/30%, for example. But my experience in helping many hundreds of men and women work with this program has been that even if they're slightly off target, missing their ratio by a percentage point or two, it doesn't make that much difference over the long term. It's much more important to stick with the program than to get the ratio absolutely perfect every time (although you always should be able to get very close).

When I placed the first clients on this program, weighing and measuring were part of the plan. I saw some of them throw up their hands in frustration—and just about throw in the towel—because of the dreadful and time-consuming task of using the scale, one meal after another. I conducted a small study that evaluated the progress made by people who relied on the scale, comparing them to a second group who went "scale-free." The result: There were no measurable differences in the success rates of the two groups. (Even so, as I'll explain later, you may find weighing and measuring food valuable as this program begins, to get a sense of what a reasonable portion of meat or milk looks like.)

Research shows that your ratios don't have to be exact down to the last decimal and percentage point. But you *do* need to pay attention to proportions and percentages when planning your meals, and you must become very aware of the specific foods and nutrient groups you need to emphasize. Always keep your own optimal ratio in mind when you're making food selections, and you'll be surprised at how close you will come—and how that is reflected in the number of pounds you lose. The sample menus later in this chapter will be key in helping you get a sense of what your food-filled plates should look like when you're eating according to your ratio. Make every meal as much on target as possible in terms of your recommended ratio.

CALORIES DO COUNT—BUT DON'T COUNT THEM!

Now, what about calories? Although calorie-counting isn't part of this program, I've taken them into account when developing this program. In this chapter, you'll find two sets of sample menus: 1,600-calories-per-day menus and 1,800-calories-per-day menus. To find out which is most appropriate for you, you need to take your ideal weight into account. Thus:

✔ If your ideal weight is 150 pounds or less (men and women), use the 1,600-calories-per-day menus.

✔ If your ideal weight is more than 150 pounds, use the 1,800-calories-per-day menus.

These are the optimal caloric-intake levels when you're trying to lose weight for the long term and enjoy lasting good health.

HOW DO YOU FEEL?

Particularly in the first few days of this program, I suggest that you monitor how you're feeling after eating. If you're uncomfortable or lethargic thirty to ninety minutes following a particular meal, it probably wasn't formulated in the ratio for which you're aiming. Your body chemistry is sending you a message that you need to do some fine-tuning. Make sure you're eating the proper proportions of nutrients in each meal for your type. On the other hand, if you're feeling alert and energetic after eating, you've probably hit the bull's-eye. Congratulations!

Remember, if you eat according to your ratio (or come very close), your body's metabolism will function optimally, you will lose weight (if that's your goal), you'll have energy and stamina that will carry you through the entire day, and your overall health will improve. You'll also develop an undeniable sense of well-being. But if you're consuming a diet with your ratios out of sync, your metabolism and other critical physiological processes will be unbalanced as well, undermining your chances of succeeding with this (or any other) program.

WHEN TO EAT—AND WHEN TO STOP

Before she began the *Metabolize* program, Martha, a woman in her late forties, was pretty fed up with weight-loss programs. "I'll tell you what I hate about diets," she said. "It's the feeling of deprivation. Nothing is worse than pushing yourself away from the dinner table and still feeling hungry! I've been on just about every diet you can think of. And I've bailed on all of them! I've always felt so deprived!"

But that wasn't the case when Martha went on *Metabolize.* You'll also discover that when you're on this program, you should never feel deprived.

Another key to making *Metabolize* work is to become very aware of your sensations of hunger and satiation. Eat when you're hungry. But stop when those hunger pangs have subsided. Don't eat beyond the point of being full or satiated.

Most people cringe when you suggest that they cut back on the amount of food they eat. Before you reject the idea, ask yourself why you eat as much as you do. You may realize that for most of your life, you've eaten for many reasons other than hunger. Eating was a social event, whether you were dining with family members or at a party. Or food gave you emotional comfort when the people in your life weren't providing it, or when you were feeling stress. Or you simply loved eating (who doesn't?), attracted by the flavors and aromas of food, and not by feelings of hunger.

I'd like you to try something different. Slow down your eating pace. After every few bites, take a brief break and ask yourself, "Am I still hungry?" If you really are, go ahead and continue eating. Enjoy your meal. Savor every bite. When you stop and ask yourself how you are feeling, however, you may discover that you're not really hungry anymore but want to continue eating for other reasons. In that case, get up from the table and move on with the rest of your day's activities. You shouldn't feel a need to finish everything on your plate—and you won't feel deprived, either, because you'll be able to eat whenever you're really hungry. You'll probably end up eating less than you usually do and lose weight in the process.

By eating slowly, you'll also get the sensors in your brain and stomach to work in harmony. Remember, your internal homeostatic system can guide you on what it needs in order to function at peak efficiency. If you're attuned to it and respond appropriately, you won't overeat. When that happens, your body will find a balance that will normalize your weight just where it should be.

PUTTING PROTEIN IN PERSPECTIVE

When it comes to high-protein foods, many of us go a little overboard. Maybe the steak that lands on our plate isn't enough to feed a family of four—but it might be close!

Here's the problem. The average person cannot digest and metabolize much more than forty grams of protein in a meal; it's just biologically impossible. And forty grams of protein really isn't that much, particularly if you're used to piling your plate high with a slab of meat about the size of the state of Vermont.

At the same time, you should be eating at least some protein with every meal. With protein present, your body burns its fuel more efficiently. Imagine, for example, an excellent grade of wood such as hard oak; if you throw gasoline and a match on it, you can expect it to burn much more slowly than cheap soft pine. In much the same way, if you were to consume carbohydrates *without* any protein, you'd burn that "fuel" rapidly, as though it were soft pine. The addition of a little protein, however, will make the fuel last longer, and your body will function much more efficiently.

How much protein should you consume in a typical meal? Ideally, think of a three-to-four-ounce portion of meat, which typically contains the target level of protein. In case you don't have a frame of reference of what three to four ounces really looks like, here's a sensible guideline that won't require you to rely on the scale: A three-to-four-ounce uncooked

Strategies for Getting Started

Once you've taken the self-test in Chapter 4 and determined your Metabolic Type and the optimal ratio (of carbohydrates, protein, and fat) for you, here are a few tips to keep in mind to help you implement the program (other suggestions appear throughout these diet-related chapters):

→ Pay close attention to the food lists for your Type, choosing from the *Preferred* foods most often, while eating items in the *Sometimes* list two or three times a week, and from the *Seldom* list only once or twice a month.

→ Follow the sample menus, particularly when you're getting started. If your ideal weight is 150 pounds or less, you should be eating 1,600 calories a day; if your optimal weight is more than 150 pounds, your target intake is 1,800 calories. Choose the sample menus accordingly.

→ Even if you aren't used to eating breakfast, make an effort to have a morning meal. Particularly for weight loss, it is best to eat (perhaps more than you're used to) early in the day, which will give you energy for the day's activities. It also minimizes cravings and maximizes fat-burning.

→ Whenever possible, select low-fat versions of the foods you put on your plate. Keep in mind, however, that low-fat items are sometimes high in calories (particularly snacks, desserts, and other processed foods), so read labels carefully.

→ Where fruits and vegetables are concerned, eat fresh or frozen whenever you can, and minimize canned or other processed varieties (although eating a canned product occasionally is better than veering off the program completely). In selecting fruit and vegetables from your food list, you can substitute fruit and vegetable juices instead; just don't overdo the amounts and keep in mind that you're consuming calories with every gulp. Keep the juices in the range of a six- to eight-ounce glass if your type is Lean or Super-Lean, a four- to six-ounce glass if you're Clean or Super-Clean, or a five- to seven-ounce glass if you're Mixed.

→ Stick to the program (and your food list) as much as possible for the next 21 days (and preferably 42 days). After six weeks, you can "stray" once in a while—having a slice of cake or a dish of ice cream if they're your favorites and even if they're not on your food list—but don't make these digressions a daily phenomenon.

serving of meat is about the size of a deck of playing cards or a closed fist. Or if you can, weigh a four-ounce portion of meat so you can get a sense of its size.

Now, what about protein-rich milk? A cup is an optimal serving size. Most people don't know what a cup of milk looks like because they are used to filling up a 16-ounce glass, and figure that's the equivalent of a cup. But a cup is eight ounces, not 16. Unless you're accustomed to thinking of eight ounces as a cup, you may have a distorted view of how much milk you should be drinking. To better acquaint you with a proper serving size, measure eight ounces of milk in a measuring cup, then pour it into your favorite glass; depending on the size of your glass, only a portion of it may be used. Keep that in mind when you drink milk and other liquids in this program.

After a while, you'll be able to "eyeball" a particular food and know approximately the portion size that's in front of you.

> **META-BITE**
>
> **C**onsume protein at every meal, and you'll efficiently use the "fuel" you consume.

VEGGIE POWER!

What's not to like about vegetables? They're very low in fat, low in calories, high in fiber, and rich in vitamins and minerals. They're also brimming with antioxidants, which are potent cancer-fighting substances.

But if you still shudder at those childhood memories of having to smother your veggies with ketchup just to make them even slightly palatable, it's time to get over it. No matter what your Metabolic Type, carbohydrates are an important part of your diet. Vegetables need to be front and center in your dietary parade.

Here are some produce pointers:

✔ When you're preparing vegetables, keep peeling and chopping to a minimum. You'll lose fewer vitamins and minerals that way.

✔ Steaming is one of the best ways to prepare vegetables. They'll be ready in just minutes and lose very little of their nutrient content and their crunchiness.

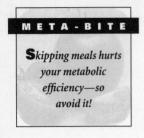

META-BITE

Skipping meals hurts
your metabolic
efficiency—so
avoid it!

✔ When stir-frying, use only small amounts of oil (one or two tablespoons). Heat the oil before placing the veggies into the pan.

✔ If you're in the habit of bathing your broccoli and other vegetables in butter, keep it under control or look for an alternative to the yellow stuff. Try seasoning veggies with a dash of curry and cayenne pepper, or perhaps Mrs. Dash seasonings. Or if you're looking for a tasty vegetable dip, try some nonfat yogurt.

DRINK UP! THE VALUE OF WATER

For *Metabolize* to work, you already know that you must pay attention to your fat-carbohydrate-protein ratio. But without plenty of water in your diet, too, this program (or any other) wouldn't make much of a ripple in improving your well-being. I recommend that you drink an eight-ounce glass of water (for example, lime water or lemon water) with or before every meal.

Here are the facts: Your body is about one-half to two-thirds water. Without water, the cells in your body could not carry out all of their life-sustaining functions. In fact, if you did not regularly replenish your body with water, you couldn't survive for more than a few days. Even though water isn't a source of energy, your body requires two to three quarts of water daily just to keep going.

Water ensures that all of the nutrients you're consuming are transported through your body, that waste removal takes place, and that all metabolic processes occur without a glitch. And while some of this water can come from your food (fruit, for example, is 80 percent water, and even lean beef is about 60 percent water), *you also need to drink six to eight glasses of water a day* to ensure that your body is awash in what it requires. It's a good idea to consume some of that water just before meals; drinking a glass each time you sit down at the dining-room table and before lifting your fork will help tame your hunger as well.

Lemon and lime water may balance the levels of body chemicals called acids and alkalis, thus preventing acidosis (above normal acidity)

More *Metabolize* Dietary Tips

As you implement the eating program for your Metabolic Type, here are additional guidelines to keep in mind:

➔ Don't concentrate solely on a small number of the foods approved for your Metabolic Type. Instead, eat a wide variety of items from the allowable list. For example, no matter what your Type, you have a dozen or more choices of seafood that fit into your eating program; try several of them in the next few weeks. You have just as many options in other food categories, including fruits and vegetables. When it comes to grains, give the more exotic ones—such as amaranth and barley—a try. Get creative with developing your own menus.

➔ Don't skip meals. Of course, some people think that the fastest way to weight loss is to avoid breakfast altogether and eat a container of yogurt for lunch. After all, they reason, that's a guaranteed way to cut down on calories. But there's plenty of research showing just how counterproductive this strategy is. When you skip meals, hunger pangs surface, and in reaction to those famished feelings, you'll be prone to so-called "rebound eating"—that is, bingeing later in the day, thus undermining your weight-loss goals. At the same time, meal skipping will downshift the internal workings of your body, slowing the metabolic rate and thus burning fewer calories, leading to *more* fat storage. Research clearly shows that the fewer meals you eat, the better your body will become at storing fat. This leads us to the following:

➔ Eat *at least* three meals a day, at approximately the same time each day. For some people, however, four, five or even six meals a day makes more sense. Let's say that you eat breakfast but are hungry, irritable, and losing energy by ten o'clock; you are probably a Super-Clean Metabolic Type and are rapidly using up that energy, as though you were pouring too much gasoline on a fire so it burned much faster than normal. In a case like this, waiting until lunchtime to eat again would be ludicrous; by then, your blood sugar levels could be completely out of kilter. And when you did finally eat lunch, if it were carbohydrate-rich (like a salad), you might be famished a short time later. If your eating pattern is like this, you should probably eat four or perhaps even five or six times a day (particularly if you feel the same letdown in midafternoon). Also, as you'll see in the sample menus, your Metabolic Type may be eating more snacks than another Type. (For example, three snacks a day are optimal for the Super-Clean metabolizers, compared to zero to one snack for the Super-Leans.)

But here's the key: If you're going to be eating four or more times per day, make sure you have smaller meals at each sitting. Initially, when you stare at your plate with a "downsized" meal on it, visions of deprivation may dance through your head. But don't forget that you'll be eating four or more times a day, not just three, and thus you'll be relishing the tastes and smells of food much more frequently. That's not exactly deprivation, is it?

If you're consuming foods in the proper ratio for your Metabolic Type, you should be able to go three to five hours between meals. But if hunger pangs and zapped energy return before three hours, consider switching to more than three meals a day. Use the sample menus in this chapter to get a sense of how much you should be eating in three meals, then divide that up among four or five meals. For example, if you're following the menus for 1,800 calories (because your ideal weight is above 150 pounds), spread out those calories over four meals, not three.

→ Minimize the salt and sugar in your diet. Although sugar may give a temporary lift to your blood sugar level, thus providing a quick burst of energy, it will dissipate rapidly, and you may develop a craving for more sugar to reenergize yourself; you might also be drawn to other unhealthy eating behaviors, since sugar cravings can lead to eating high-fat foods to satisfy yourself. A better way to keep your energy levels *consistently* high is to eat a balanced diet in the nutrient ratio aligned with your Metabolic Type. It will provide a more gradual increase in blood sugar levels—and they're more likely to stay high rather than taking a rapid dive. So stamp out sugar whenever you can, and don't forget the blizzard of foodstuffs in which sugar may be hidden. When sugar is added to processed food, it might be called sucrose, dextrose, fructose, corn syrup, or malt. There's nothing sweet about that.

As for salt, remember that if you overdo it, salt promotes fluid retention in your tissues. This buildup of fluid can trigger not only weight gain but potentially serious problems such as high blood pressure, kidney stones, and osteoporosis (a bone-thinning disease). My advice: Remove the salt shaker from your dining-room table, and use salt sparingly during cooking; learn to enjoy the natural flavors of food. Choose fresh, unprocessed foods whenever possible, but if you buy packaged foods, read the labels carefully, and shy away from high-sodium items. Also, keep in mind that many dairy products tend to be high in sodium; a cup of some brands of cottage cheese, for example, may have as much sodium as more than 60 potato chips!

→ Don't forget about other spices and condiments that you may routinely add to your food. Avoid croutons on your salad. Use salad dressings with care, since even the nonfat variety can still be high in calories and sugar. Try enhancing the flavor of your salads (as well as vegetables) with natural herbs.

in the muscle tissue that causes everything from joint problems to mood swings. Many people become too acidic because of the wheat and high-protein meats they consume, but the right fruits and vegetables—and especially lime or lemon water with meals—can keep your acid and alkali levels in balance.

You don't need to choose the fanciest lime-flavored bottled water on the supermarket shelves. Adding lime or lemon to mineral water, sparkling water, club soda, spring water, seltzer, and the latest fad drinks is fine, but in nearly all communities, simple tap water will make just as big a splash. By law, tap water has to meet the Environmental Protection Agency's safety standards, although if you live in a rural community, make some inquiries to ensure that the well water has been properly tested and won't cause health problems. Because of copper pipes, some tap water may cause toxic reactions in people sensitive to copper. If you have any concerns about your own city's water supply, consider installing a water filter on your kitchen faucet. But remember, the formula for water is pretty simple—two parts hydrogen to one part oxygen. That is its composition, no matter where it comes from.

What if your taste buds rebel when you drink tap water? That's the case with me. I simply don't like the taste of the chlorine in the tap water in my own community. For that reason, I personally rely on bottled water. But if tap water satisfies your taste buds, it will quench the requirements of this program.

What about carbonated drinks? They're high in either sugar or artificial sweeteners, and while they might satisfy your sweet tooth, they have no real nutritional value. To make matters worse, many soft drinks contain plenty of phosphorus, which interferes with the body's ability to use calcium.

I've saved the best about water for last. It is calorie-free. So if weight loss is your goal, drink as much water as you want, and don't worry about a tidal wave of calories dampening your efforts.

CHANGE IS ON THE WAY

Once you've altered the way you eat, brace yourself for some dramatic changes. Most of them, of course, will be positive—but initially, some of them may actually be unpleasant. In the first few days of eating in support of your Metabolic Type, your body may stage something of a mini-insurrection, rebelling against the transformation underway. You might experience headaches, perhaps some stomach upsets, and then you might feel tired. In a real sense, your system is undergoing detoxification. You may be eating properly for the first time in your life, and your body needs to clean itself out—a first step toward feeling much better.

Don't panic. Most people start feeling fine, usually within 24 to 48 hours. But you may be one of those whose system requires a little extra time, maybe four to seven days, particularly if you've been a heavy caffeine or sugar user. To make the process a little easier, concentrate more on consuming fruits and vegetables and their juices, while eating fewer grains.

Stick with it. Any unpleasant moments will be short-lived, and then it will be smooth sailing. Amazingly, once you get your ratios right and without any extra work, your metabolic efficiency will improve and your weight will automatically move in the direction of your optimal level. After I adopted the diet for my Type (Mixed), I lost 25 pounds, without any effort toward changing my calorie intake (although I did avoid junk food) and while still eating to satisfaction. Just altering the ratios—making sure I was eating fats, proteins and carbohydrates in the proper combinations—made the difference.

Of course, calories can't be ignored. But 1,600 calories of lettuce isn't the same as 1,600 calories of beef. You'll burn them for fuel differently. You'll metabolize them differently. So with your Metabolic Type in mind, what you eat is as important as the number of calories you consume.

As your body chemistry changes, you too will start to shed the pounds that may have stubbornly hung on to your frame for years. All of the little embarrassments that are part of weighing more than you'd like—including feeling the emotional pain of cruel comments about your size—will melt away as rapidly as your extra weight does. Your clothes will fit better, you will feel lighter and be able to move with more ease, you will experience less stress on the joints, and you'll have more energy than you've had in years. (Check your driver's license; you might feel younger than you really are!) You'll be in control of your health and your life, experience more emotional balance, and probably start enjoying each day a lot more. And by taking better care of yourself today, you'll pave the way for a healthier tomorrow, too.

BEFORE YOU START

Prior to eating in accordance with your Metabolic Type, here's a valuable exercise that I recommend. For three days, keep a food diary of what you normally eat and how you feel in the hour or two after your meals. Be honest. Don't leave anything out just because you're writing it down. Eat the way you always do to satisfy your hunger and cravings. This exercise will give you a clear sense of what you've been eating and how it affects your well-being. Use the accompanying tables for this purpose.

DAY 3 BEFORE *METABOLIZE*

Foods Eaten Today _____
(date)

BREAKFAST:

_____

_____

_____

_____

After eating breakfast today, my general feeling of well-being had the following rating on a 1 to 5 point scale (with 1 representing feeling tired or run-down, and 5 representing feeling great).

1   2   3   4   5   *(circle one)*

LUNCH:

_____

_____

_____

_____

After eating lunch today, my general feeling of well-being had the following rating on a 1 to 5 point scale (with 1 representing feeling tired or run-down, and 5 representing feeling great).

1   2   3   4   5   *(circle one)*

DINNER:

_____

_____

_____

_____

After eating dinner today, my general feeling of well-being had the following rating on a 1 to 5 point scale (with 1 representing feeling tired or run-down, and 5 representing feeling great).

1   2   3   4   5   *(circle one)*

DAY 2 BEFORE *METABOLIZE*

Foods Eaten Today _____
(date)

BREAKFAST:

_____

_____

_____

_____

After eating breakfast today, my general feeling of well-being had the following rating on a 1 to 5 point scale (with 1 representing feeling tired or run-down, and 5 representing feeling great).

1   2   3   4   5   *(circle one)*

LUNCH:

_____

_____

_____

_____

After eating lunch today, my general feeling of well-being had the following rating on a 1 to 5 point scale (with 1 representing feeling tired or run-down, and 5 representing feeling great).

1   2   3   4   5   *(circle one)*

DINNER:

_____

_____

_____

_____

After eating dinner today, my general feeling of well-being had the following rating on a 1 to 5 point scale (with 1 representing feeling tired or run-down, and 5 representing feeling great).

1   2   3   4   5   *(circle one)*

DAY 1 BEFORE *METABOLIZE*

Foods Eaten Today _____
(date)

BREAKFAST:

_____

_____

_____

_____

After eating breakfast today, my general feeling of well-being had the following rating on a 1 to 5 point scale (with 1 representing feeling tired or run-down, and 5 representing feeling great).

1   2   3   4   5   *(circle one)*

LUNCH:

_____

_____

_____

_____

After eating lunch today, my general feeling of well-being had the following rating on a 1 to 5 point scale (with 1 representing feeling tired or run-down, and 5 representing feeling great).

1   2   3   4   5   *(circle one)*

DINNER:

_____

_____

_____

_____

After eating dinner today, my general feeling of well-being had the following rating on a 1 to 5 point scale (with 1 representing feeling tired or run-down, and 5 representing feeling great).

1   2   3   4   5   *(circle one)*

SAMPLE MENUS

This section provides a series of menus to help you implement the dietary program for your own Metabolic Type. For each Type, I've provided seven days of menus—that is, three meals a day plus snacks for a total of seven days—for two calorie intakes. The meals are relatively simple, designed to make it as easy as possible for you to get started with this plan. They will also help you see how to create your own menus, using the food lists in Chapter 5, to fit the ratio assigned to your Type.

If your ideal weight is 150 pounds or less, choose from the 1,600-calories-a-day menus; if your ideal weight is over 150 pounds, select from the 1,800-calories-a-day menus.

At the end of the menus for each Metabolic Type, I've provided a nutritional breakdown of the calories and grams of carbohydrates, fat, and protein for each meal; these are the targets you should be aiming for when you create menus of your own.

Over the course of this program, I encourage you to eat a wide variety of foods from your own food list. With this approach, you'll more rapidly reach your goals of feeling and looking better, attaining your ideal body weight, and achieving optimal health.

1,600-CALORIES-A-DAY MENUS

SUPER-LEAN

70% CARBOHYDRATES / 15% PROTEIN / 15% FAT

BREAKFAST 1	☙ EGGS
	3 egg whites
	1 oz. Soyrizo
	½ pat butter (slightly less than 1 tsp.)
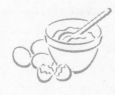	
	☙ TORTILLA
	1 sprouted wheat tortilla
	PREPARATION: On one side of a pan, scramble eggs with nonfat cooking spray; on the other side, add Soyrizo, mash into small chunks, and cook. When eggs are almost done, mix together. Warm the

tortilla, add ½ pat butter. Serve with mango and pineapple chunks.

❧ FRUIT
1 mango
1 cup pineapple chunks

BREAKFAST 2

❧ YOGURT
1 cup low-fat yogurt
½ oz. English walnuts

❧ FRUIT
1 kiwi
1 papaya
2 figs

BREAKFAST 3

❧ SOY DREAM AND CEREAL
1 cup multigrain cereal (sprouted preferred)
POUR ON: *¾ cup vanilla Soy Dream*
TOP WITH: *2 strawberries (sliced)*

❧ SOY DREAM, STRAWBERRY AND BANANA
1 cup vanilla Soy Dream
BLEND WITH:
⅓ banana
2 strawberries

BREAKFAST 4

❧ OATMEAL
1 cup oatmeal (cooked according to package directions)
1 cup skim milk (add desired amount to oatmeal; drink the rest)
MIX WITH:
1 tbsp. raisins
1½ tsp. almonds (or 5 whole)
cinnamon to taste

⊷ **10 CHERRIES**

BREAKFAST 5

⊷ **TOFU SCRAMBLE**

3 oz. firm tofu*
¼ green pepper (chopped)
¼ red pepper (chopped)
1 tsp. chopped onion
pinch of cilantro
pinch of garlic
slice of lime
2 tbsp. salsa
½ oz. low-fat cheddar cheese (grated)
½ sprouted wheat tortilla

PREPARATION: Scramble tofu in a pan sprayed with nonfat cooking spray. When nearly done, add peppers, onion, cilantro, garlic, lime, and salsa. Top with cheese. Use the tortilla for dipping, or place the tofu in it and turn it into a burrito.

⊷ **FRUIT BOWL**

1 plum
15 cherries
15 grapes
1 cup casaba melon cubes
2 cups watermelon cubes

BREAKFAST 6

⊷ **SPECIAL K CEREAL**

1½ cups Special K cereal
WITH:
1 cup 1% milk
¼ cup blackberries
1½ tsp. slivered almonds (or 5 whole)

---

*A variety of tofu dishes and seasonings are appropriate for the *Metabolize* plan, such as tofu versions of chow mein and stroganoff. Brand names include Tofu Mate and Fantastic Classics. (Gluten-free products are preferred.)

❧ **FRUIT**
½ pink grapefruit
1 pear

BREAKFAST 7

❧ **WHEAT BREAD**
1 slice sprouted wheat bread (toasted)
1 tbsp. reduced-fat peanut butter

❧ **FRUIT**
1 plum
½ papaya

❧ **KEFIR**
1 cup reduced-fat kefir

LUNCH 1

❧ **FISH**
2½ oz. white fish, broiled or baked
SEASONINGS: *lemon, paprika, parsley*

❧ **PASTA**
1 cup artichoke pasta (cooked)
2 tsp. olive oil
1 carrot (thickly sliced)
½ cup green peas
½ clove garlic (minced)
Italian seasoning to taste
PREPARATION: Cook pasta according to package directions. In a separate pan, heat olive oil; then add carrot, peas, and garlic. Heat and tenderize. Add pasta. Mix well and serve warm.

LUNCH 2	**❧ BURGER DELUXE** *1 Boca burger* *2 slices sprouted sourdough bread (toasted)* WITH: 　*1 tbsp. lite mayonnaise* 　*mustard or ketchup to taste* *1 leaf romaine lettuce* *1 slice onion* *1 slice tomato* **❧ FRUIT** *1 pear* *3 apricots*

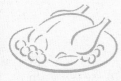

LUNCH 3	**❧ SOUTHWESTERN CHICKEN SALAD** *2½ oz. chicken breast (skinless, boneless)* *½ cup assorted dried fruit* *⅛ cup black beans (cooked)* *1 oz. jicama (diced)* *1 oz. scallions (minced)* *1 tsp. lite mayonnaise* *1 tbsp. lite sour cream* *1 tsp. crushed red pepper flakes* PREPARATION:

1. Place chicken in a saucepan with water and boil. (Or if you prefer, grill the chicken.) Cook until tender. Then cut chicken into ½-inch pieces.
2. Bring water in a pan to a boil. Add dried fruit slowly, keeping the water boiling. Boil for 10 minutes, stirring once or twice. Drain, rinse in cold water. Drain again.
3. Combine all ingredients, including the chicken, and toss to mix thoroughly. Cover and chill for at least 2 hours.
4. Serve slightly chilled.

⤙ FRUIT
¾ mango

LUNCH 4

⤙ TUNA SANDWICH
2 oz. Bumble Bee white tuna in water
1 tbsp. lite mayonnaise
⅛ stalk celery (chopped)
2 black olives (chopped)
lemon pepper
dash of lemon juice
2 slices sprouted wheat bread (toasted)
alfalfa sprouts
PREPARATION: Mix tuna, mayonnaise, celery, olives, pepper, and juice. Serve on toast with sprouts.

⤙ RICE
¼ cup cooked basmati rice

⤙ FRUIT
1 apple
2 prunes

LUNCH 5

⤙ COTTAGE CHEESE
½ cup 1% cottage cheese
1 slice pineapple

⤙ VEGETABLE DISH
1 cup mixed vegetables (broccoli, corn, red peppers)
⅓ package Arrowhead wild rice and herbs
3 cashews (chopped)
PREPARATION: Cook vegetables and rice separately. Then mix together, and add cashews.

LUNCH 6

❧ TURKEY SANDWICH
2 oz. turkey (seasoned)
2 slices sprouted sourdough bread
2 tsp. lite mayonnaise
Dijon mustard to taste
1 leaf lettuce

❧ FRUIT
1 pear
1 apple

LUNCH 7

❧ COBB SALAD
3 leaves iceberg lettuce
4 leaves romaine lettuce
1 hard-boiled egg sliced; (use only ½ yolk)
1 hard-boiled egg white
1 oz. low-fat Colby cheese (grated)
2 mushrooms (sliced)
1 radish (sliced)
2 black olives (sliced)
¼ carrot (sliced)
alfalfa sprouts
2 tsp. Weight Watchers creamy ranch dressing
PREPARATION: Tear lettuce leaves into bite sizes, and place in bowl. Add all other ingredients.

❧ BAKED POTATO
6 oz. baked potato with skin
   (if no skin, add 1 Ry-Krisp to meal)
2 tbsp. lite sour cream or 1 pat butter
   SEASON WITH: *salt substitute*

DINNER 1

❧ **BEAN AND BARLEY STEW**

¼ cup pinto beans (dry)
¼ cup Eden organic adzuki beans (dry)
½ cup pearled barley
1 cup low-sodium vegetable broth
1 celery stalk (in chunks)
½ parsnip (peeled and sliced)
½ tbsp. minced onion
1 tsp. olive oil
pepper to taste
salt substitute to taste
Cholula to taste
2 tsp. chopped fresh sage (or ½ tsp. dried sage)
½ sweet potato (peeled and diced)

PREPARATION: Rinse, soak overnight, and cook according to each package's directions. Cook barley according to package instructions. In a large pot, combine beans with barley, vegetable broth, and 1 cup of cold water. Also add celery, parsnip, onion, olive oil, sweet potato, and seasonings. Bring to boil, then simmer for 12 to 15 minutes or until tender.

DINNER 2

❧ **TURKEY MOZZARELLA**

2 oz. turkey breast
1½ tsp. olive oil
½ cup spaghetti sauce
1½ tsp. vinegar
1 cup spinach spaghetti (cooked)
1 oz. Almond Rella mozzarella cheese

PREPARATION: Cook and brown turkey breast in olive oil. Add spaghetti sauce and vinegar. Serve over spaghetti, topped with cheese.

↝ SALAD

¼ head iceberg lettuce (bite-size pieces)

¼ head romaine lettuce (bite-size pieces)

1 carrot (sliced)

1 celery stalk (sliced)

1 radish (sliced)

¼ cucumber (sliced)

1 tbsp. minced red onion

COMBINE FOR DRESSING:

1½ tsp. olive oil

1½ tsp. balsamic vinegar

Italian seasoning to taste

DINNER 3

↝ VEGETABLE-BASIL RICE

1 cup Arrowhead quick wild rice and herbs

½ cup frozen peas

¼ carrot (diced)

¼ cup sliced green onions

1 oz. firm tofu

1 tsp. olive oil

1 tsp. low-sodium soy sauce

pinch of garlic

PREPARATION: Prepare rice according to directions on package. Cook vegetables and tofu in olive oil, soy sauce, and garlic until tender. Mix in rice.

↝ SIDE DISHES

¾ cup green beans (steamed)

10 grapes

DINNER 4

↝ COD

2½ oz. baked Atlantic cod

SEASONINGS: lime, cilantro to taste

❧ BEAN DISH

¾ cup cooked pinto beans
1 tsp. garlic
1 tsp. diced jalapeño pepper
Cholula sauce to taste
1 tbsp. mashed avocado
2 corn tortillas
PREPARATION: Simmer the pinto beans, adding the garlic, jalapeño, and Cholula sauce. Add the avocado when serving. Use the tortillas for dipping.

❧ SALAD

¼ head romaine lettuce (bite-size pieces)
4 leaves spinach (bite-size pieces)
4 broccoli flowerettes
1 tbsp. chopped red onion
sprinkle of alfalfa sprouts
COMBINE FOR DRESSING:
1 tsp. olive oil
1 tsp. balsamic vinegar or to taste

❧ SIDE DISH

1 nectarine
4 oz. pineapple juice drink

DINNER 5

❧ QUICK CHILI

¼ Boca burger
1 cup Hidden Valley mild vegetarian chili
1 sprouted wheat tortilla
1 pat butter
PREPARATION: Crumble Boca burger, fry, and add it to chili. Serve with buttered tortilla.

❧ FRUIT

1 papaya

DINNER 6

❖ **GRILLED PINEAPPLE-TERIYAKI CHICKEN**

2 oz. chicken breast
1 pineapple ring
1 tbsp. teriyaki sauce

PREPARATION: Grill chicken breast; when one side is done, turn over, top with pineapple and sauce. Cook until done.

❖ **SIDE DISHES**

1 cup Lipton Golden fried rice, cooked according to package directions
1½ cups green beans (steamed)
1 pat butter (to taste)
season to taste

DINNER 7

❖ **MACADAMIA AND PINEAPPLE RICE PILAF**

1 pat butter
½ cup long-grain white rice (uncooked)
½ clove garlic (minced)
¼ red bell pepper (cut into matchsticks)
¼ yellow pepper (cut into matchsticks)
1 cup canned reduced-fat vegetable broth
1 tbsp. golden raisins
3 oz. lite firm tofu
½ cup diced pineapple
1 tbsp. cilantro
2 macadamia nuts (chopped)

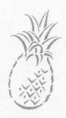

PREPARATION: In a pan, melt butter, and add rice. Stir frequently until rice is lightly browned. Add garlic and peppers, stirring frequently for 1 minute. Add broth; bring to boil. Reduce heat to low, add raisins, cover, and simmer for 20 minutes. Stir-fry tofu separately; break up tofu, and then add pineapple, cilantro, macadamia nuts, and rice mixture. Season to taste.

SIDE DISH

¾ cup Horizon fat-free yogurt

SNACK

CHOOSE 0 OR 1 PER DAY

- 5 oz. Soy Dream Vanilla Light
  4 grapes

- 4 oz. Soy Dream Chocolate Light

- 3 Ry-Krisp
  1 oz. Rice Slices cheddar/American cheese (melt over Ry-Krisp)
  1 plum

- Metabolize™ Nutri-Shake (as directed on label)*

- ½ Metabolize™ Nutri-Bar*

- Smoothie
  BLEND:
    4 oz. orange juice
    ½ cup pineapple (fresh, frozen, or canned in own juice)
    ½ scoop whey protein powder
  ADD: *½ tsp. olive oil*

- 1 peach
  1 fig
  1 oz. Almond Rella mozzarella cheese

- reduced-fat strawberry kefir (just under ½ cup)

*For sources of Metabolize™ products: *www.metabol:2e.net* or 1-800-828-3343

SUPER-LEAN: NUTRITIONAL BREAKDOWN (1,600 CALORIES)		
Breakfast, Lunch, and Dinner (500 calories each)		
Carbohydrate:	350 calories	87 grams
Protein:	75 calories	19 grams
Fat:	75 calories	8 grams
Snack (100 calories)		
Carbohydrate:	70 calories	17 grams
Protein:	15 calories	4 grams
Fat:	15 calories	2 grams

LEAN

60% CARBOHYDRATES / 20% PROTEIN / 20% FAT

BREAKFAST 1	❖ **EGGS AND TORTILLA** *4 egg whites* *1½ oz. Soyrizo* *1 sprouted wheat tortilla* *½ pat butter* PREPARATION: On one side of pan, scramble egg whites with nonstick cooking spray; on the other side, add Soyrizo, mash into small chunks, and cook. When eggs are almost done, mix the two together. Serve on warm tortilla, with ½ pat butter. ❖ **FRUIT** *1 mango* *½ pineapple ring*
BREAKFAST 2	❖ **TURKEY SAUSAGE** *½ Shelton's organic turkey sausage patty* PREPARATION: Fry in pan with a little water.

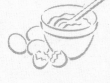

↝ **YOGURT DISH**
1 cup low-fat yogurt
3 walnut halves, crushed
¼ cup blueberries

↝ **FRUIT**
1 kiwi
1 papaya
1 fig

BREAKFAST 3

↝ **SOY DREAM AND CEREAL**
1 cup sprouted multigrain cereal
    POUR ON: *¾ cup vanilla Soy Dream*
    TOP WITH: *2 sliced strawberries*

↝ **SOY DREAM, STRAWBERRY, AND BANANA**
1 cup vanilla Soy Dream
    BLEND WITH:
    ½ scoop whey protein powder
    2 strawberries
    1 banana
    ADD: *Water to thin, if needed*

BREAKFAST 4

↝ **OATMEAL**
1 cup oatmeal (cooked)
1 cup skim milk (add desired amount to oatmeal;
    drink the rest)

↝ **TOAST**
1 slice sprouted wheat bread (toasted)
1 tbsp. reduced-fat peanut butter (spread on toast)

BREAKFAST 5

❧ TOFU SCRAMBLE
3 oz. firm tofu*
¼ green pepper (chopped)
¼ red pepper (chopped)
1 tsp. chopped onion
pinch of cilantro
pinch of garlic
squeeze of lime
2 tbsp. salsa
1 oz. low-fat cheddar cheese (grated)
1 sprouted wheat tortilla
PREPARATION: Scramble tofu in a pan. When nearly cooked, add peppers, onion, cilantro, garlic, lime, and salsa. Top with cheese. Use the tortilla for dipping, or place the tofu in it and turn it into a burrito.

❧ FRUIT BOWL
8 cherries
8 grapes
1 cup casaba melon cubes
2 cups watermelon cubes

BREAKFAST 6

❧ SPECIAL K CEREAL
1½ cups Special K cereal
   WITH:
      1 cup 2% milk
      2 tbsp. blackberries
      1 tsp. raisins
      1 tsp. slivered almonds (or 3 whole)

*A variety of tofu dishes and seasonings are appropriate for the *Metabolize* plan, such as tofu versions of chow mein and stroganoff. Brand names include Tofu Mate and Fantastic Classics. (Gluten-free products are preferred.)

◦ **SAUSAGE**
1 Garden sausage (cooked according to package directions)

BREAKFAST 7

◦ **GARDEN SAUSAGE**

◦ **WHEAT BREAD**
1 slice sprouted wheat bread (toasted)
1 tbsp. reduced-fat peanut butter

◦ **FRUIT**
1 plum

◦ **KEFIR**
1 cup reduced-fat kefir
⅓ scoop whey protein (blend with kefir)

LUNCH 1

◦ **FISH**
3 oz. white fish (broiled or baked)
   SEASONINGS: *lemon, paprika, parsley*

◦ **PASTA**
1 cup artichoke pasta (cooked)
2½ tsp. olive oil
½ carrot (thickly sliced)
¼ cup green peas
½ clove garlic (minced)
Italian seasoning to taste
PREPARATION: Cook pasta according to package directions. In a separate pan, heat olive oil; then add carrot, peas, and garlic, and cook until tender. Add pasta. Mix well and serve warm.

LUNCH 2

◦ **BURGER DELUXE**
1 Boca burger
1 slice Rice Slices American cheese
2 slices sprouted sourdough bread (toasted)

WITH:

1 tbsp. lite mayonnaise

mustard or ketchup to taste

1 leaf romaine lettuce

1 slice onion

1 slice tomato

❖ FRUIT

1 pear

3 apricots

LUNCH 3

❖ SOUTHWESTERN CHICKEN SALAD

3½ oz. chicken breast (skinless, boneless)

⅓ cup assorted dried fruit

⅛ cup cooked black beans

1 oz. jicama (diced)

1 oz. scallions (minced)

1 tsp. lite mayonnaise

1 tbsp. sour cream

1 tsp. crushed red pepper flakes

PREPARATION:

1. Place chicken in a saucepan with water and boil. (Or if you prefer, grill the chicken.) Cook until tender. Then cut chicken into ½-inch pieces.
2. Bring water in a pan to a boil. Add dried fruit slowly, keeping the water boiling. Boil for 10 minutes, stirring once or twice. Drain, rinse in cold water. Drain again.
3. Combine all ingredients, including the chicken, and toss to mix thoroughly. Cover and chill for at least 2 hours.
4. Serve slightly chilled.

❦ **FRUIT**
¾ mango

LUNCH 4

❦ **TUNA SANDWICH**
3 oz. Bumble Bee white tuna in water
1 tbsp. lite mayonnaise
⅛ stalk celery (chopped)
2 black olives (chopped)
lemon pepper to taste
dash of lemon juice
2 slices sprouted wheat bread (toasted)
alfalfa sprouts
PREPARATION: Mix tuna, mayonnaise, celery, olives, pepper, and juice. Serve on toast with sprouts.

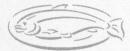

❦ **RICE**
¼ cup cooked basmati rice
½ pat butter (add to rice)

❦ **FRUIT**
1 apple

LUNCH 5

❦ **COTTAGE CHEESE**
¾ cup 1% cottage cheese

❦ **VEGETABLE DISH**
¾ cup mixed vegetables (broccoli, corn, red peppers)
⅓ package Arrowhead wild rice and herbs
3 crushed cashews
PREPARATION: Cook vegetables and rice separately. Then mix together, and add cashews.

LUNCH 6	◆ **TURKEY SANDWICH** 2½ oz. turkey (seasoned) 2 slices sprouted sourdough bread 1 tbsp. lite mayonnaise Dijon mustard 1 leaf lettuce 1 tomato slice ◆ **FRUIT** 1 pear ½ apple
LUNCH 7 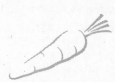	◆ **COBB SALAD** 3 leaves iceberg lettuce 4 leaves romaine lettuce 1 hard-boiled egg (sliced) 2 hard-boiled egg whites (sliced) 1 oz. low-fat Colby cheese (grated) 2 mushrooms (sliced) 1 radish (sliced) 2 olives (sliced) ¼ carrot (sliced) alfalfa sprouts 2 tsp. Weight Watchers creamy ranch dressing PREPARATION: Tear lettuce leaves into bite sizes and place in bowl. Add all other ingredients. ◆ **BAKED POTATO** 6 oz. baked potato with skin 　(if no skin, add 1 Ry-Krisp to meal) 2 tbsp. lite sour cream (and chives) or 1 pat butter 　SEASON WITH: salt substitute to taste

DINNER 1

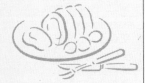

✧ **BEAN AND BARLEY STEW**

¼ cup pinto beans (dry)
¼ cup Eden organic adzuki beans (dry)
1 cup low-sodium vegetable broth
1 oz. beef eye of round
¼ cup pearled barley
1 celery stalk (in chunks)
½ parsnip (peeled and sliced)
1 tbsp. minced onion
2 tsp. olive oil
pepper to taste
salt substitute to taste
Cholula to taste
2 tsp. chopped fresh sage (or ½ tsp. dried sage)

PREPARATION: Rinse, soak overnight, and cook according to each package's directions. Cook barley according to package instructions. In a large pot, combine beans with barley, vegetable broth and 1 cup of cold water. Brown beef, and add beef, barley, celery, parsnip, onion, olive oil, and seasonings. Bring to boil, then simmer for 12 to 15 minutes or until tender.

DINNER 2

✧ **TURKEY MOZZARELLA**

2½ oz. turkey breast (diced)
½ cup spaghetti sauce
1 cup spinach spaghetti (cooked)
1 oz. Almond Rella mozzarella cheese

PREPARATION: Cook and brown turkey breast in olive oil. Serve over cooked spaghetti topped with spaghetti sauce and cheese.

✦ SALAD

¼ head iceberg lettuce

¼ head romaine lettuce

1 carrot (sliced)

1 celery stalk (sliced)

1 radish (sliced)

¼ cucumber (sliced)

1 tbsp. minced red onion

COMBINE FOR DRESSING:

2 tsp. olive oil

2 tsp. balsamic vinegar

Italian seasoning to taste

DINNER 3

✦ VEGETABLE-BASIL RICE

1 cup Arrowhead quick wild rice and herbs

½ cup frozen peas

¼ carrot (sliced)

¼ cup sliced green onions

3 oz. firm tofu

2 tsp. olive oil

1 tbsp. low-sodium soy sauce

pinch of garlic

PREPARATION: Prepare rice according to directions on package. Cook vegetables and tofu in olive oil, soy sauce, and garlic until tender. Mix in rice.

✦ FRUIT

5 grapes

DINNER 4

✦ BAKED COD

3 oz. Atlantic cod (baked)

SEASONINGS: lime, cilantro to taste

- **BEAN DISH**
¾ *cup cooked pinto beans*
1 tsp. garlic
1 tsp. diced jalapeño pepper
Cholula sauce to taste
2 tbsp. mashed avocado
2 corn tortillas
PREPARATION: Simmer the pinto beans, adding the garlic, jalapeño, and Cholula sauce. Add the avocado when serving. Use the tortillas for dipping.

- **SALAD**
¼ head romaine lettuce (bite-size pieces)
4 leaves spinach (bite-size pieces)
4 broccoli flowerettes
1 tbsp. chopped red onion
sprinkle of alfalfa sprouts
COMBINE FOR DRESSING:
1 tsp. olive oil
1 tsp. balsamic vinegar or to taste

- **SIDE DISH**
4 oz. pineapple juice drink

DINNER 5

- **QUICK CHILI**
½ Boca burger
1 cup Hidden Valley mild vegetarian chili
1 sprouted wheat tortilla
1 pat butter
PREPARATION: Crumble Boca burger, fry, and add it to chili. Serve with buttered tortilla.

- **FRUIT AND CHEESE**
½ papaya
1 slice Rice Slices American cheese

DINNER 6

GRILLED PINEAPPLE-TERIYAKI CHICKEN

3 oz. chicken breast
1 pineapple ring
1 tbsp. teriyaki sauce

PREPARATION: Grill chicken breast; when one side is done, turn over, top with pineapple and sauce. Cook until done.

SIDE DISHES

1 cup Lipton Golden fried rice cooked according to package directions
½ cup green beans (steamed)
season to taste

DINNER 7

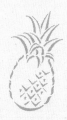

MACADAMIA AND PINEAPPLE RICE PILAF

1 pat butter
½ cup long-grain white rice (uncooked)
½ clove garlic (minced)
¼ red bell pepper (cut into matchsticks)
¼ yellow pepper (cut into matchsticks)
2 cups canned reduced-fat vegetable broth
1 tbsp. golden raisins
3 oz. chicken breast
½ cup diced pineapple
1 tbsp. cilantro
1 macadamia nut (chopped)

PREPARATION: In a pan, melt butter, and add rice. Stir frequently until rice is lightly browned. Add garlic and peppers, stirring frequently for 1 minute. Add broth; bring to boil. Reduce heat to low, add raisins, cover, and simmer for 20 minutes. Boil or grill chicken. Dice. Add chicken, pineapple, cilantro, and nut to rice mixture. Season to taste.

SNACKS	❧ (CHOOSE 1 OR 2 PER DAY)

- 8 oz. Vitasoy Carob Supreme*

- 2 Ry-Krisp
  1 oz. Rice Slices cheese (melted over Ry-Krisp)
  1 plum

- Metabolize™ Nutri-Shake (as directed on label)**

- ½ Metabolize™ Nutri-Bar**

- Smoothie
  BLEND:
  4 oz. orange juice
  ⅓ cup pineapple (fresh, frozen, or canned in own juice)
  ⅓ scoop whey protein powder

- 3 almonds

- 1 peach
  1 oz. Almond Rella mozzarella cheese

LEAN: NUTRITIONAL BREAKDOWN (1,600 CALORIES)		
Breakfast, Lunch, and Dinner (500 calories each)		
Carbohydrate:	300 calories	75 grams
Protein:	100 calories	25 grams
Fat:	100 calories	11 grams
Snack (100 calories)		
Carbohydrate:	60 calories	15 grams
Protein:	20 calories	5 grams
Fat:	20 calories	2 grams

*Available in most health food stores and some supermarkets.
**For sources of Metabolize™ products: *www.metabolize.net* or 1-800-828-3343

MIXED

50% CARBOHYDRATES / 25% PROTEIN / 25% FAT

BREAKFAST 1	**AMERICAN SCRAMBLE** *1 whole egg* *2 egg whites* *1½ pats butter* *salt substitute to taste* *1 Garden sausage* *1 slice sprouted wheat bread (toasted)* *1 tbsp. ketchup (optional)* PREPARATION: Scramble eggs in ½ pat butter, season with favorite salt substitute. Top with ketchup if desired. Fry sausage according to package directions, using a nonfat cooking spray. Serve with toast and 1 pat butter. **FRUIT** *15 grapes*
BREAKFAST 2	**BREAKFAST SALAD** *⅞ cup regular cottage cheese* *1 apple (cored, sliced)* *1 peach (pitted, sliced)* *¾ cup pineapple (chunks)* *1 walnut half (chopped)*
BREAKFAST 3	**QUICK BREAKFAST** *6 oz. grape juice (100%, no sugar added)* *¾ banana* *1¼ scoops whey protein powder* *1 tsp. olive oil* *4 ice cubes (optional)* *3 macadamia nuts* PREPARATION: In blender, mix all ingredients, except nuts. Eat nuts separately.

BREAKFAST 4	❧ OATMEAL
	½ cup oatmeal (cooked)
	WITH:
	½ cup 1% milk
	1 tsp. slivered almonds
	1 tsp. raisins
	sprinkle of cinnamon (to taste)
	❧ BACON
	2½ oz. Canadian bacon
	PREPARATION: Fry bacon in nonfat cooking spray.
	❧ FRUIT
	10 cherries
BREAKFAST 5	❧ MEXICAN SCRAMBLE
	1 whole egg
	3 egg whites
	½ tsp. olive oil
	2 tbsp. salsa
	1 oz. low-fat cheddar cheese (grated)
	pinch of cilantro
	PREPARATION: Scramble eggs in olive oil. When almost done, add salsa, cheese, and cilantro.
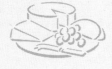	
	❧ TORTILLA
	1 sprouted whole wheat tortilla
	❧ FRUIT
	2 plums

BREAKFAST 6	❖ **BREAKFAST STEAK** *2 oz. breakfast steak (lean beef)* PREPARATION: Broil steak; season to taste. ❖ **SPECIAL K CEREAL** *1 cup Special K* *¾ cup vanilla Soy Dream (pour on cereal)* ❖ **FRUIT** *1 kiwi*
BREAKFAST 7 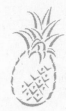	❖ **FRUIT NUT YOGURT** *1 cup low-fat yogurt* *1 cup pineapple chunks* *1 cup watermelon chunks* *2 tbsp. slivered almonds* PREPARATION: Mix yogurt, fruit, and almonds together. ❖ **SAUSAGE** *2½ oz. Louis Rich turkey sausage* PREPARATION: Prepare according to package directions.
LUNCH 1	❖ **CHEESEBURGER** *3 oz. extra lean ground beef* *2 tsp. diced onion* *1 tsp. Worcestershire sauce* *1 slice Healthy Choice American cheese* *1 leaf lettuce* *1 slice tomato* *ketchup and mustard to taste* *2 slices rye or sprouted wheat bread (toasted)* PREPARATION: Mix beef, onion, and Worcestershire sauce together. Broil or grill; add cheese when nearly done. Top with lettuce, tomato, and condiments; serve on toast.

◆ **FRUITS AND NUTS**
1 Asian pear
10 grapes
4 cashews

LUNCH 2

◆ **GRILLED SALMON**
3 oz. Atlantic salmon
lemon, paprika, parsley to taste
PREPARATION: Squeeze lemon over salmon while grilling. Sprinkle with paprika and parsley.

◆ **SIDE DISHES**
⅓ cup basmati rice (cooked)
1 cup broccoli (steamed)
TOPPED WITH: *1 pat butter*

LUNCH 3

◆ **TURKEY SANDWICH**
2 oz. turkey breast
1 slice Alpine Lace reduced-fat Swiss cheese
2 slices rye or sprouted wheat bread
1 tbsp. mayonnaise
1 slice tomato
1 leaf lettuce

◆ **FRUIT**
1 plum
1 apple
5 grapes

LUNCH 4

◆ **CHICKEN STIR-FRY**
2½ oz. chicken breast (sliced)
⅓ cup pea pods
¼ red pepper (cut into matchsticks)
¼ green pepper (cut into matchsticks)
1 tsp. yellow onion (chopped)
¼ cup zucchini (cut into matchsticks)

1 clove garlic (minced)

2¼ tsp. olive oil

2 tbsp. low-sodium soy sauce

1 cup brown rice (cooked)

PREPARATION: Broil or grill chicken. Dice and set aside. Stir-fry vegetables in oil until tender. Add chicken and soy sauce to vegetables, and heat through. Spoon over warm rice.

LUNCH 5

TUNA SANDWICH

3 oz. chunky white tuna in water (drained)

½ stalk celery (chopped)

2 tbsp. lite mayonnaise

2 slices sprouted wheat bread (toasted if desired)

1 leaf lettuce

1 slice tomato

1 black olive (chopped)

PREPARATION: Mix tuna, celery, mayonnaise, and olive together, and place on bread. Top with lettuce and tomato.

FRUIT

1 apple

LUNCH 6

BEEF FAJITA

3 oz. eye of round beef (sliced)

½ lime

1 package dry fajita mix (reduced to serving size)

¼ red pepper (cut into matchsticks)

¼ yellow pepper (cut into matchsticks)

2 tsp. Spanish onion (chopped)

1 sprouted wheat tortilla

1½ tbsp. guacamole

PREPARATION: Brown the beef in nonfat cooking spray or water, and drain. Squeeze lime over beef. Add fajita mix, and cook according to package directions. Steam vegetables separately. Assemble fajita with wheat tortilla, and top with guacamole.

◆ BEAN DISH
¾ cup pinto beans (cooked)
1 tsp. diced jalapeños
PREPARATION: Heat beans with jalapeños. (If preferred, omit jalapeños and season to taste.)

LUNCH 7

◆ SUPER SALAD
4 leaves romaine lettuce
2 leaves Bibb lettuce
2 leaves spinach
1 hard-boiled egg (chopped)
2 hard-boiled egg whites (chopped)
2 oz. chicken breast (grilled, broiled, or boiled, then chopped)
½ tomato (cut in wedges)
1 tsp. red onion (minced)
4 broccoli flowerettes
4 cauliflower flowerettes
1 carrot (sliced)
1 tbsp. enoki mushrooms (diced)
1 radish (sliced)
2 tbsp. Weight Watchers creamy ranch dressing
PREPARATION: Tear lettuce leaves into bite-size pieces, and place in a bowl. Combine with other ingredients.

◆ CELERY STALKS
2 celery stalks (whole)
2 tbsp. peanut butter (place on stalks)

DINNER 1

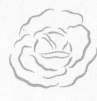

❧ BAKED CHICKEN
½ tsp. paprika
¼ tsp. curry powder
pinch oregano
pinch white pepper
1 chicken leg and thigh (bone-in, skinless)
PREPARATION: Mix seasonings in plastic bag. Shake well. Coat chicken with bag's contents. Spray butter-flavored, nonfat cooking spray on baking dish. Bake covered at 350° for 25 to 30 minutes, or until juices run clear.

❧ SALAD
3 leaves romaine lettuce
3 leaves spinach
1 tomato (wedges)
1 stalk celery (chopped)
1 tbsp. red onion (diced)
1 radish (sliced)
2 tbsp. Weight Watchers creamy cucumber dressing
PREPARATION: Tear lettuce leaves into bite-size pieces. Combine all ingredients.

❧ BLACK-EYED PEAS
¼ cup black-eyed peas (cook according to package directions)
1 tsp. nonfat bacon bits
ALTERNATIVE: Prepare a can of Allen's black-eyed peas with bacon.

❧ FRUIT
½ cup sliced cling peaches (in heavy syrup)

DINNER 2	**⚘ STEAK** *3½ oz. top sirloin (lean and fat-trimmed)* *1 tbsp. A•1 steak sauce or favorite seasonings* PREPARATION: Grill or broil steak. Season with steak sauce or seasonings. **⚘ VEGETABLE SIDE DISHES** 1 cup green beans (steamed) SEASON WITH: 　*1 clove garlic (minced)* 1 small sweet potato (baked) 1 raw carrot 1½ pats butter
DINNER 3	**⚘ BROILED COD** *3½ oz. Pacific cod* *1 lemon wedge* *1 pat butter (melted)* *paprika and parsley to taste* PREPARATION: Squeeze lemon on cod and set aside for 5 minutes. Pour melted butter over cod. Sprinkle with paprika and parsley. Broil. **⚘ BARLEY DISH** *⅔ cup barley* *1 pat butter* *Mrs. Dash or favorite seasoning* PREPARATION: Cook barley according to package directions. Add butter and seasoning. **⚘ SIDE DISH** *1 peach* *5 black cherries* *3 cashews*

DINNER 4	❧ **SPAGHETTI WITH MEAT SAUCE** *3 oz. ground beef (extra lean)* *Italian seasoning to taste* *½ cup Healthy Choice spaghetti sauce* *¾ cup spinach spaghetti (cooked)* PREPARATION: Brown ground beef, drain fat, and rinse under hot water. Season. Pour sauce into skillet or saucepan, add seasoned meat, and simmer. Pour over cooked spaghetti. ❧ **BREAD** *1 slice sprouted sourdough bread (toasted if desired)*

DINNER 5	❧ **MARINATED FLANK STEAK**
	3 oz. flank steak
	  MARINADE:
	    1 tbsp. minced chipotle chili
	    1 tsp. minced garlic
	    1 tbsp. chopped cilantro
	    ½ tsp. olive oil
	    1 tbsp. soy sauce
	PREPARATION: Place flank steak in baking dish. Combine marinade ingredients and pour over steak. Turn steak over to coat well. Cover and refrigerate for 4 hours. Broil or grill until done.
	
	❧ **GREEN PEA DISH**
	¾ cup green peas
	2 cauliflower flowerettes
	1 small carrot (sliced)
	1 tsp. onion (chopped)
	Mrs. Dash or other salt substitute
	PREPARATION: Steam or boil vegetables. Season to taste.

❧ BARLEY DISH

4 cauliflower flowerettes
½ cup barley (cooked)
Mrs. Dash or other salt substitute to taste.

DINNER 6

❧ GRILLED SALMON

3 oz. salmon (grilled)
lemon and paprika, to taste
PREPARATION: Squeeze lemon on salmon while grilling. Sprinkle with paprika.

❧ ASPARAGUS SIDE DISH

4 asparagus spears
½ pat butter

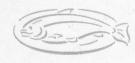

❧ QUINOA SIDE DISH

⅓ cup quinoa
⅔ cup water
1 tsp. olive oil
1 tbsp. lemon juice
½ clove garlic (minced)
1 celery stalk (diced)
1 tbsp. yellow onion (chopped)
¼ cup red pepper (chopped)
parsley to taste
½ tomato (diced)
PREPARATION: Cook quinoa according to package directions. Heat olive oil and garlic in skillet. Then add celery, onion, red pepper, parsley, and tomato. Sauté until tender. Add lemon juice. Mix in quinoa.

DINNER 7

◆ BAKED CORNISH HEN

1 Cornish hen
1 tbsp. tahini butter
1 clove garlic (minced)
pepper to taste
favorite salt substitute to taste
juice of 1 lemon

PREPARATION: Rinse hen and place, breast side down, on work surface. With kitchen shears, split lengthwise along backbone. Turn hen over, and press down with your palm to flatten breastbone. Remove skin from hen. Score meat at 1-inch intervals. Place in baking dish. Rub both sides with tahini butter. Sprinkle with garlic, seasonings, and lemon juice. Cover and refrigerate for 1 hour. Roast breast side down at 425 degrees for 15 minutes; turn over and continue roasting for another 15 minutes or until juices run clear. Eat all of hen except for half of one breast.

◆ VEGETABLE DISH

4 broccoli flowerettes
4 slices cucumber
2 celery sticks
3 green olives
2 tomato slices
1 carrot

◆ RICE DISH

⅔ cup wild rice

PREPARATION: Cook according to package directions. Season with favorite salt substitute, if desired.

SNACKS	❧ (CHOOSE 2 PER DAY)

- 2 oz. Rice Slices American cheese
  1 apple

- ⅓ cup 2% cottage cheese
  2 celery stalks
  1½ tsp. cashew butter (place on celery stalks)
  2 small carrots

- Metabolize™ Nutri-Bar*

- Metabolize™ Nutri-Shake*

- ⅔ cup low-fat yogurt
  ½ tsp. slivered almonds
  6 black cherries (crushed)

PREPARATION: Mix almonds and cherries into yogurt.

- Smoothie
  BLEND:
  4 oz. orange juice
  ⅓ cup pineapple chunks
  ½ scoop whey protein powder

  4 almonds

- 2 Ry-Krisp
  1½ oz. turkey (white or dark meat)
  2 macadamia nuts
  6 cherries

*For sources of Metabolize™ products: *www.metabolize.net* or
1-800-828-3343

MIXED: NUTRITIONAL BREAKDOWN (1,600 CALORIES)		
Breakfast (400 calories)		
Carbohydrate:	200 calories	50 grams
Protein:	100 calories	25 grams
Fat:	100 calories	11 grams
Lunch and Dinner (450 calories each)		
Carbohydrate:	225 calories	56 grams
Protein:	112 calories	28 grams
Fat:	112 calories	12 grams
Snack (150 calories x 2)		
Carbohydrate:	75 calories	19 grams
Protein:	37 calories	9 grams
Fat:	37 calories	4 grams

CLEAN

40% CARBOHYDRATES / 30% PROTEIN / 30% FAT

BREAKFAST 1

 AMERICAN SCRAMBLE

1 egg

3 egg whites

1½ pats butter

favorite salt substitute to taste

1 tbsp. ketchup (optional)

1 Garden sausage

1 slice sprouted wheat bread (toasted)

PREPARATION: Scramble eggs in ½ pat butter; season. Top with ketchup if desired. Fry sausage according to package directions, using a nonfat cooking spray. Serve with toast and 1 pat butter.

 FRUIT

5 grapes

BREAKFAST 2	◆ BREAKFAST SALAD *1 cup regular cottage cheese* *1 apple (cored, sliced)* *1 peach (pitted, sliced)* *3 walnut halves (chopped)*
BREAKFAST 3	◆ QUICK BREAKFAST *¾ cup grape juice (100%, no sugar added)* *⅔ banana* *1½ scoops whey protein* *1 tsp. olive oil* *4 ice cubes (optional)* *4 macadamia nuts* PREPARATION: In blender, mix all ingredients except nuts. Eat nuts separately.

BREAKFAST 4	◆ OATMEAL
	½ cup oatmeal (cooked)
	   WITH:
	     1 cup 1% milk
	     2 tsp. slivered almonds (or 6 whole almonds)
	     2 tsp. raisins
	     sprinkle of cinnamon (to taste)
	
	◆ BACON
	2½ oz. Canadian bacon
	PREPARATION: Fry bacon in nonfat cooking spray or cook in water.

BREAKFAST 5

❧ **MEXICAN SCRAMBLE**
1 egg
3 egg whites
1 tsp. olive oil
2 tbsp. salsa
1 oz. low-fat cheddar cheese (grated)
pinch of cilantro
PREPARATION: Scramble eggs in olive oil. When almost done, add salsa, cheese, and cilantro.

❧ **TORTILLA**
1 sprouted wheat tortilla

❧ **FRUIT**
1 plum

BREAKFAST 6

❧ **BREAKFAST STEAK**
3 oz. breakfast steak (extra lean)
PREPARATION: Broil steak; season to taste.

❧ **SPECIAL K CEREAL**
1 cup Special K
¾ cup vanilla Soy Dream (place on cereal)

BREAKFAST 7

❧ **FRUIT NUT YOGURT**
1¼ cups low-fat yogurt
1 cup pineapple chunks
½ cup watermelon chunks
1 tsp. slivered almonds (or 3 whole almonds)
PREPARATION: Mix yogurt, fruit, and almond together.

❧ **SAUSAGE**
2½ oz. Louis Rich turkey sausage
PREPARATION: Prepare according to package directions.

LUNCH 1	❧ **CHEESEBURGER**

3½ oz. ground beef (extra lean)
2 tsp. diced onion
1 tsp. Worcestershire sauce
1 slice Healthy Choice American cheese
1 leaf lettuce
1 slice tomato
2 slices rye or sprouted wheat bread (toasted)
ketchup and mustard to taste
PREPARATION: Mix beef, onion, and Worcestershire sauce. Shape into burger, and broil or grill. Add cheese when nearly done. Top with lettuce and tomato. Serve on toast with condiments to taste.

❧ **FRUIT**
1 Asian pear

LUNCH 2   ❧ **GRILLED SALMON**
4 oz. Atlantic salmon
lemon, paprika, parsley to taste
PREPARATION: Squeeze lemon over salmon while grilling. Sprinkle with paprika and parsley.

❧ **SIDE DISHES**
• ¼ cup basmati rice (cooked)
• 1 cup broccoli (steamed)
TOPPED WITH: *1 pat butter*

LUNCH 3   ❧ **TURKEY SANDWICH**
3 oz. turkey breast
1 slice Alpine Lace reduced-fat Swiss cheese
2 slices rye or sprouted wheat bread
1½ tbsp. lite mayonnaise
1 slice tomato
1 leaf lettuce

❖ **FRUIT**
1 plum
6 grapes

LUNCH 4

❖ **CHICKEN STIR-FRY**
3½ oz. chicken breast
¼ cup pea pods
¼ red pepper (cut into matchsticks)
¼ green pepper (cut into matchsticks)
2 tsp. chopped yellow onion
¼ cup zucchini (cut into matchsticks)
1 clove garlic (minced)
1 tbsp. olive oil
2 tbsp. low-sodium soy sauce
1 cup brown rice (cooked)
PREPARATION: Boil or grill chicken. Dice and set aside. Stir-fry vegetables in oil until tender. Add chicken and soy sauce to vegetables, and heat through. Spoon over warm rice.

LUNCH 5

❖ **TUNA SANDWICH**
4 oz. chunky white tuna in water (drained)
½ stalk celery (chopped)
2 tbsp. lite mayonnaise
2 slices sprouted wheat bread (toasted if desired)
1 leaf lettuce
1 slice tomato (optional)
3 black olives (chopped)
PREPARATION: Mix tuna, celery, mayonnaise, and olives together, and place on bread. Top with lettuce and tomato.

❖ **FRUIT**
¾ apple

LUNCH 6

❧ **BEEF FAJITA**

4 oz. eye of round beef (sliced)
½ lime
1 package dry fajita mix (reduced to serving size)
¼ red pepper (cut into matchsticks)
¼ yellow pepper (cut into matchsticks)
2 tsp. diced Spanish onion
1 sprouted wheat tortilla
2 tbsp. guacamole
PREPARATION: Brown the beef in nonfat cooking spray or water; drain. Squeeze lime over beef. Add fajita mix, and cook according to package directions. Steam vegetables separately. Assemble fajita with wheat tortilla, and top with guacamole.

❧ **BEAN DISH**

¼ cup pinto beans (cooked)
1 tsp. diced jalapeños
PREPARATION: Heat beans with jalapeños. (If preferred, omit jalapeños and season to taste.)

LUNCH 7

❧ **SUPER SALAD**

4 leaves romaine lettuce
2 leaves Bibb lettuce
2 leaves spinach
1 hard-boiled egg (chopped)
2 hard-boiled egg whites (chopped)
2½ oz. chicken breast (grilled, broiled, or boiled,
    then chopped)
½ tomato (cut in wedges)
1 tsp. diced red onion
4 cauliflower flowerettes
1 carrot (sliced)
1 tbsp. enoki mushrooms (diced)
4 black olives (sliced)
1 radish (sliced)
2 tbsp. Weight Watchers creamy ranch dressing

PREPARATION: Tear lettuce leaves into bite sizes, and place in a bowl. Add all other ingredients.

❖ **CELERY STALKS**
2 celery stalks
1 tbsp. peanut butter (place on celery stalks)

DINNER 1

❖ **BAKED CHICKEN**
½ tsp. paprika
¼ tsp. curry powder
pinch oregano
pinch white pepper
1 chicken leg and thigh (bone-in, skinless)
PREPARATION: Mix seasonings in plastic bag. Shake well. Coat chicken with bag's contents. Spray butter-flavored, nonfat cooking spray on baking dish. Bake covered at 350° for 25 to 30 minutes, or until juices run clear.

❖ **SALAD**
3 leaves romaine lettuce
3 leaves spinach
1 tomato (wedges)
1 stalk celery (chopped)
1 tbsp. diced red onion
1 radish (sliced)
1 tsp. sunflower seeds
2 tbsp. Weight Watchers creamy cucumber dressing
PREPARATION: Tear lettuce leaves into bite sizes. Combine all ingredients.

⟜ BLACK-EYED PEAS

*½ cup black-eyed peas (cooked according to package
    directions)*
1 tsp. nonfat bacon bits
ALTERNATIVE: Prepare a can of Allen's black-eyed
peas with bacon.

DINNER 2

⟜ STEAK

4 oz. top sirloin (lean and fat-trimmed)
1 tbsp. A•1 steak sauce or favorite seasonings
PREPARATION: Grill or broil steak. Season with
steak sauce or seasonings.

⟜ VEGETABLE SIDE DISHES

1 cup green beans (steamed)
SEASON WITH:
  ½ pat butter
  1 clove garlic (minced)
1 small sweet potato (baked)
SEASON WITH:
  *1 pat butter (or 1½ pats, if you leave the butter
    off the green beans)*

DINNER 3

⟜ BROILED COD

4½ oz. Pacific cod
1 lemon wedge
1 pat butter (melted)
paprika and parsley to taste
PREPARATION: Squeeze lemon on cod, and set
aside for 5 minutes. Pour melted butter over cod.
Sprinkle with paprika and parsley. Broil.

❧ BARLEY DISH
½ cup barley
1 pat butter
Mrs. Dash or favorite seasoning
PREPARATION: Cook barley according to package directions. Add butter and seasoning.

❧ FRUIT
1 peach
6 black cherries
6 cashews

DINNER 4

❧ SPAGHETTI WITH MEAT SAUCE
4 oz. ground beef (extra lean)
Italian seasoning to taste
½ cup Healthy Choice spaghetti sauce
⅔ cup spinach spaghetti (cooked)
PREPARATION: Brown ground beef, drain fat, and rinse under hot water. Season. Place sauce in skillet or saucepan, add seasoned beef, and simmer. Pour over cooked spaghetti.

❧ BREAD
1 slice sprouted sourdough bread (toasted if desired)

DINNER 5

❧ MARINATED FLANK STEAK
5 oz. flank steak
   MARINADE:
      1 tbsp. minced chipotle chili
      1 tsp. minced garlic
      1 tbsp. chopped cilantro
      1 tsp. olive oil
      1 tbsp. soy sauce
PREPARATION: Place steak in baking dish. Combine marinade ingredients, and pour over steak. Turn steak over to coat well. Cover and refrigerate for 4 hours. Broil or grill until done.

❧ GREEN PEA DISH
½ cup green peas
1 tsp. onion (chopped)
Mrs. Dash or other salt substitute
PREPARATION: Steam or boil vegetables. Season.

❧ BARLEY DISH
½ cup barley (cooked)
Mrs. Dash or other salt substitute to taste

DINNER 6

❧ GRILLED SALMON
3½ oz. salmon (grilled)
lemon and paprika to taste
PREPARATION: Squeeze lemon on salmon while grilling. Sprinkle with paprika.

❧ ASPARAGUS SIDE DISH
4 asparagus spears (steamed)
   WITH: *½ pat butter*

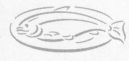

❧ QUINOA SIDE DISH
⅓ cup quinoa
½ cup water
1 tsp. olive oil
½ clove garlic (minced)
1 celery stalk (diced)
1 tbsp. yellow onion (chopped)
¼ cup chopped red pepper
½ tomato (diced)
parsley to taste
PREPARATION: Cook quinoa according to package directions. Heat olive oil and garlic in skillet. Then add celery, onion, red pepper, parsley, and tomato. Sauté until tender. Mix in quinoa.

DINNER 7

⚬ BAKED CORNISH HEN

1 Cornish hen
1 tbsp. tahini butter
juice of 1 lemon
1 clove garlic (minced)
pepper to taste
favorite salt substitute to taste

PREPARATION: Rinse hen and place, breast side down, on work surface. With kitchen shears, split lengthwise along backbone. Turn hen over, and press down with your palm to flatten breastbone. Remove skin from hen. Score meat at 1-inch intervals. Place in baking dish. Rub both sides with tahini butter. Sprinkle with lemon juice, garlic, and seasonings. Cover and refrigerate for 1 hour. Roast breast side down at 425 degrees for 15 minutes; turn over and continue roasting for another 15 minutes or until juices run clear.

⚬ VEGETABLE DISH

4 slices cucumber
2 celery sticks
3 green olives
2 tomato slices

⚬ RICE DISH

1 cup wild rice

PREPARATION: Cook according to package directions. If desired, flavor with favorite salt substitute.

SNACKS	❧ (CHOOSE 2 PER DAY)

- 1 oz. reduced fat cheddar cheese
  ½ apple

- ⅓ cup low-fat cottage cheese
  2 celery stalks
  2 tsp. cashew butter (place on celery stalks)

- Metabolize™ Nutri-Bar*

- Metabolize™ Nutri-Shake*

- ¾ cup low-fat yogurt
  1 tsp. slivered almonds (or 3 whole)
  4 black cherries (crushed)

  PREPARATION: Mix almonds and cherries into yogurt.

- 1 hard-boiled egg
  1 hard-boiled egg white
  15 grapes

- 1½ oz. turkey
  ¾ pear
  2 macadamia nuts

- ⅓ cup low-fat cottage cheese
  1 cup chopped walnuts
  ½ cup pineapple chunks

- 1½ oz. chicken (coated with 1 tsp. mayonnaise and pepper)
  1¼ cup watermelon cubes

*For sources of Metabolize™ products: *www.metabolize.net* or 1-800-828-3343

CLEAN: NUTRITIONAL BREAKDOWN (1,600 CALORIES)		
Breakfast (400 calories)		
Carbohydrate:	160 calories	40 grams
Protein:	120 calories	30 grams
Fat:	120 calories	13 grams
Lunch and Dinner (450 calories each)		
Carbohydrate:	180 calories	45 grams
Protein:	135 calories	34 grams
Fat:	135 calories	15 grams
Snack (2 snacks; 150 calories each)		
Carbohydrate:	60 calories	15 grams
Protein:	45 calories	11 grams
Fat:	45 calories	5 grams

SUPER-CLEAN

35% CARBOHYDRATES / 35% PROTEIN / 30% FAT

BREAKFAST 1

 AMERICAN SCRAMBLE

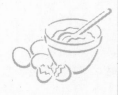

1 egg
3 egg whites
1½ pats butter
favorite salt substitute to taste
1 tbsp. ketchup (optional)
1 Boca sausage
1 slice sprouted wheat bread (toasted)

PREPARATION: Scramble eggs in ½ pat butter; season with salt substitute. Top with ketchup if desired. Fry sausage in nonfat cooking spray or cook in a little water. Serve with toast and 1 pat butter.

 FRUIT

½ cup natural sliced cling peaches (in own juice)

BREAKFAST 2	✦ BREAKFAST SALAD
	1¼ cups regular cottage cheese
	1 apple (cored, sliced)
	½ peach (pitted, sliced)
	2 walnut halves (chopped)
BREAKFAST 3	✦ QUICK BREAKFAST
	¾ cup grape juice (100%, no sugar added)
	½ banana
	1¾ scoops whey protein
	1 tsp. olive oil
	4 ice cubes (optional)
	3 macadamia nuts
	PREPARATION: Blend all ingredients, except nuts. Eat nuts separately.
BREAKFAST 4	✦ OATMEAL
	½ cup oatmeal (cooked)
	WITH:
	¾ cup 1% milk
	1½ tsp. slivered almonds
	1 tsp. raisins
	sprinkle of cinnamon to taste
	✦ BACON
	3 oz. Canadian bacon
	PREPARATION: Fry bacon in nonfat cooking spray.
	✦ EGG
	1 egg (hard boiled or soft boiled)
BREAKFAST 5	✦ MEXICAN SCRAMBLE
	1 egg
	4 egg whites
	1 tsp. olive oil

2 tbsp. salsa
1 oz. low-fat cheddar cheese (grated)
pinch of cilantro
PREPARATION: Scramble eggs in olive oil. When almost done, add salsa, cheese, and cilantro.

❖ **TORTILLA**
1 whole sprouted wheat tortilla

❖ **FRUIT**
½ plum

BREAKFAST 6

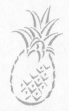

❖ **BREAKFAST STEAK**
3½ oz. breakfast steak
PREPARATION: Broil steak; season to taste.

❖ **SPECIAL K CEREAL**
⅔ cup Special K
⅔ cup vanilla Soy Dream (place on cereal)

BREAKFAST 7

❖ **FRUIT NUT YOGURT**
1¼ cups low-fat yogurt
1 pineapple ring
1 cup watermelon cubes
1 tsp. slivered almonds (or 3 whole)
PREPARATION: Mix yogurt, fruit, and almonds.

❖ **SAUSAGE**
3½ oz. Louis Rich turkey sausage
PREPARATION: Prepare according to package instructions.

LUNCH 1

❖ **CHEESEBURGER**
4 oz. ground beef (extra lean)
2 tsp. diced onion
1 tsp. Worcestershire sauce

1 slice Healthy Choice American cheese
1 leaf lettuce
1 slice tomato
2 slices rye or sprouted wheat bread (toasted)
ketchup and mustard to taste
PREPARATION: Mix beef, onion, and Worcestershire sauce. Shape into patty, and broil or grill. Add cheese when nearly done. Top with lettuce and tomato. Serve on toast with condiments.

❧ **FRUIT**
½ Asian pear

LUNCH 2

❧ **GRILLED SALMON**
5 oz. Atlantic salmon
lemon, paprika, parsley to taste
PREPARATION: Grill salmon. Squeeze lemon over fish. Sprinkle with paprika and parsley.

❧ **SIDE DISHES**
- ¼ cup basmati rice (cooked)
- ¾ cup broccoli (steamed)
  TOPPED WITH: *1 pat butter*

LUNCH 3

❧ **TURKEY SANDWICH**
4 oz. turkey breast
1 slice Alpine Lace reduced-fat Swiss cheese
2 slices rye or sprouted wheat bread
1½ tbsp. mayonnaise
1 slice tomato
1 leaf lettuce

❧ **FRUIT**
1 plum

LUNCH 4	✦ CHICKEN STIR-FRY

4½ oz. chicken breast (sliced)
¼ cup pea pods
¼ red pepper (diced)
1 tsp. chopped yellow onion
¼ cup matchstick-cut zucchini
1 clove garlic (minced)
2½ tsp. olive oil
2 tbsp. low-sodium soy sauce
¾ cup brown rice (cooked)
PREPARATION: Broil or grill chicken. Set aside. Sauté vegetables in oil until tender. Add chicken and soy sauce to vegetables, and mix. Serve over rice.

LUNCH 5

✦ TUNA SANDWICH
5 oz. chunky white tuna in water
2 tbsp. lite mayonnaise
2 slices sprouted wheat bread (toasted if desired)
1 leaf lettuce
1 tomato slice (optional)
3 black olives (chopped)
PREPARATION: Mix tuna and mayonnaise together, and place on bread. Top with lettuce and olives (or eat olives separately).

✦ FRUIT
1 peach

| LUNCH 6 | ❧ BEEF FAJITA |

5 oz. eye of round beef (sliced)
½ lime
1 package dry fajita mix (reduced to serving size)
¼ red pepper (cut in matchsticks)
¼ yellow pepper (cut in matchsticks)
2 tsp. diced Spanish onion
1 sprouted wheat tortilla
1½ tbsp. guacamole

PREPARATION: Brown the beef in nonfat cooking spray, and drain. Squeeze lime over beef. Add fajita mix, and cook according to package directions. Steam vegetables separately. Assemble fajita with wheat tortilla, and top with guacamole.

❧ FRUIT
⅓ papaya

| LUNCH 7 | ❧ SUPER SALAD |

4 leaves romaine lettuce
2 leaves Bibb lettuce
2 leaves spinach
1 hard-boiled egg (chopped)
3 hard-boiled egg whites (chopped)
2½ oz. chicken breast (grilled, broiled, or boiled, then chopped)
½ tomato (cut in wedges)
1 tsp. minced red onion
2 cauliflower flowerettes
½ carrot (sliced)
1 tbsp. enoki mushrooms (diced)
4 black olives (sliced)
1 radish (sliced)

PREPARATION: Tear lettuce leaves into bite-size pieces, and place in a bowl. Add all other ingredients.

❖ **CELERY STALKS**
2 celery stalks
1 tbsp. peanut butter (place on stalks)

DINNER 1

❖ **BAKED CHICKEN**
½ tsp. paprika
¼ tsp. curry powder
pinch oregano
pinch white pepper
1 chicken leg and thigh (bone-in, skinless)
PREPARATION: Mix seasonings in plastic bag. Shake well. Coat chicken with bag's contents. Spray butter-flavored, nonfat cooking spray on baking dish. Bake chicken, covered at 350° for 25 to 30 minutes, or until juices run clear.

❖ **SALAD**
3 leaves romaine lettuce
3 leaves spinach
2 hard-boiled egg whites
½ tomato (chunks)
1 tbsp. diced red onion
1 radish (sliced)
1 tsp. sunflower seeds
2 tbsp. Weight Watchers creamy cucumber dressing
PREPARATION: Tear lettuce leaves into bite sizes. Combine all ingredients.

❖ **BLACK-EYED PEAS**
½ cup black-eyed peas (cooked according to directions on can)
1 tsp. nonfat bacon bits
ATERNATIVE: Prepare a can of Allen's black-eyed peas with bacon, according to directions and use ½ cup in this dish.

DINNER 2	❦ **STEAK**
	5 oz. top sirloin (lean and fat-trimmed)
	1 tbsp. A•1 steak sauce or favorite seasonings
	PREPARATION: Grill or broil steak, and season with steak sauce or seasonings.

❦ **VEGETABLE SIDE DISHES**
½ cup green beans (steamed)
FLAVOR WITH:
1 clove garlic (minced)

1 sweet potato (baked)
FLAVOR WITH:
1 pat butter

| **DINNER 3** | ❦ **BROILED COD** |

5½ oz. Pacific cod
1 lemon wedge
1 pat butter (melted)
paprika and parsley to taste
PREPARATION: Squeeze lemon on cod, and set aside for 5 minutes. Pour melted butter over cod. Sprinkle with paprika and parsley. Broil.

❦ **BARLEY DISH**
½ cup barley (uncooked)
1 pat butter
Mrs. Dash or favorite seasoning
PREPARATION: Cook barley according to package instructions. Add butter and seasoning.

❦ **FRUIT AND NUTS**
1 peach
6 cashews

DINNER 4	**❧ SPAGHETTI WITH MEAT SAUCE**

5 oz. ground beef (extra lean)
Italian seasoning to taste
½ cup Healthy Choice spaghetti sauce
⅔ cup spinach spaghetti (cooked)

PREPARATION: Brown the ground beef, drain fat, and rinse under hot water. Season. Place sauce in a skillet or saucepan, add beef, and simmer. Pour over cooked spaghetti.

❧ BREAD

¾ slice sprouted sourdough bread (toasted if desired)

DINNER 5

❧ MARINATED FLANK STEAK

5 oz. flank steak
    MARINADE:
        1 tbsp. minced chipotle chili
        1 tsp. minced garlic
        1 tbsp. chopped cilantro
        1 tsp. olive oil
        1 tbsp. soy sauce

PREPARATION: Place steak in baking dish. Combine marinade ingredients, and pour over steak. Turn steak over to coat well. Cover and refrigerate for 4 hours. Broil or grill until done.

❧ VEGETABLE DISH

½ cup green peas
2 cauliflower flowerettes
1 tsp. chopped onion
Mrs. Dash or other salt substitute to taste

PREPARATION: Steam or boil (in a little water) the vegetables. Season.

❧ **BARLEY DISH**
⅓ cup barley (cooked)
Mrs. Dash or other salt substitute to taste

DINNER 6

❧ **GRILLED SALMON**
4½ oz. salmon (grilled)

❧ **ASPARAGUS SIDE DISH**
8 asparagus spears
  WITH: ½ pat butter

❧ **QUINOA SIDE DISH**
¼ cup quinoa
½ tsp. olive oil
½ clove garlic (minced)
1 celery stalk (sliced)
1 tsp. yellow onion (chopped)
¼ cup red pepper (chopped)
parsley to taste
1 tomato (sliced)

PREPARATION: Cook quinoa according to package instructions. Heat olive oil and garlic in skillet. Then add celery, onion, red pepper, parsley, and tomato. Sauté until tender. Mix in quinoa.

DINNER 7

❧ **BAKED CORNISH HEN**
1½ Cornish hens
1 tbsp. tahini butter
1 clove garlic (minced)
pepper to taste
favorite salt substitute to taste
juice of 1 lemon

PREPARATION: Rinse hen and place, breast side down, on work surface. With kitchen shears, split lengthwise along backbone. Turn hen over and press down with your palm to flatten breastbone. Remove skin from hen. Score meat at 1-inch intervals. Place in baking dish. Rub both sides with tahini butter. Sprinkle with garlic, seasonings, and lemon juice. Cover and refrigerate for 1 hour. Roast breast side down at 425 degrees for 15 minutes; turn over and continue roasting for another 15 minutes or until juices run clear.

✤ VEGETABLE DISH
4 slices cucumber
2 green olives
2 tomato slices
1 carrot

✤ RICE DISH
⅔ cup wild rice (uncooked)
PREPARATION: Cook according to package instructions.

SNACKS

✤ (CHOOSE 3 PER DAY)
- 1½ oz. lowfat cheddar cheese
  ½ apple

- ⅓ cup low-fat cottage cheese (1%)
  ¾ peach
  1 celery stalk
  1 tsp. cashew butter (place on celery stalk)

- Metabolize™ Nutri-Bar*

- Metabolize™ Nutri-Shake*

- ½ cup low-fat yogurt

*For sources of Metabolize™ products: *www.metabolize.net* or 1-800-828-3343

1 tsp. slivered almonds
4 black cherries (crushed)
PREPARATION: Mix almonds and cherries into yogurt.

- 1 hard-boiled egg (omit ½ egg yolk)
  1 hard-boiled egg white
  ½ cup grapes (about 10 grapes)

- 1½ oz. turkey
  ⅓ pear
  1½ macadamia nuts

- ½ cup low-fat yogurt
  1 tsp. crushed or slivered cashews (or 2 whole)
  3 pineapple chunks

- 1½ oz. chicken (coated with 2 tsp. lite mayonnaise and pepper)
  ⅔ cup watermelon cubes

SUPER-CLEAN: NUTRITIONAL BREAKDOWN (1,600 CALORIES)		
Breakfast (400 calories)		
Carbohydrate:	140 calories	35 grams
Protein:	140 calories	35 grams
Fat:	120 calories	13 grams
Lunch and Dinner (450 calories each)		
Carbohydrate:	157.5 calories	39 grams
Protein:	157.5 calories	39 grams
Fat:	135 calories	15 grams
Snack (3 snacks; 100 calories each)		
Carbohydrate:	35 calories	9 grams
Protein:	35 calories	9 grams
Fat:	30 calories	3 grams

1,800-CALORIES-A-DAY MEALS

If you're eating according to the 1,800-calories-a-day plan, your menus are not much different than those of the 1,600-calorie program. In fact, the primary meals (breakfast, lunch, dinner) remain the same; you will increase only the number and/or content of the snacks. That's all that's going to change.

So for your three main meals each day, refer to the 1,600-calorie menus for your Metabolic Type in the preceding pages. Then, rather than following the snack recommendations in those sections, adopt the snacks below for your Metabolic Type. They will add 200 calories a day to your total intake, and bring you up to your 1,800-calories-a-day target.

SUPER-LEAN

SNACKS	❧ (CHOOSE 0 OR 1 PER DAY)
	• 1 cup Soy Dream Vanilla 1 banana
	• 1¼ cups Soy Dream Chocolate
	• 1 oz. chicken breast 1 oz. Rice Slices American Cheese 1 mango 4 Ry-Krisp 2 tsp. almond butter PREPARATION: Melt cheese over chicken; spread almond butter on Ry-Krisp.
	• Metabolize™ Nutri-Bar*
	• Metabolize™ Nutri-Shake*
	• Smoothie BLEND: *1 cup orange juice* *½ cup pineapple chunks* *½ banana*
	*For sources of Metabolize™ products: *www.metabolize.net* or 1-800-828-3343

½ scoop whey protein
8 almonds

- 1 pear
  1 fig
  1 peach
  7 cherries
  2½ oz. Almond Rella mozzarella cheese

SUPER-LEAN: NUTRITIONAL BREAKDOWN (1,800 CALORIES)		
Breakfast, Lunch, and Dinner (500 calories each)		
Carbohydrate:	350 calories	87 grams
Protein:	75 calories	19 grams
Fat:	75 calories	8 grams
Snack (300 calories)		
Carbohydrate:	210 calories	52 grams
Protein:	45 calories	11 grams
Fat:	45 calories	5 grams

LEAN

SNACKS   ❖ (CHOOSE 1 OR 2 PER DAY)
- 1½ cups Soy Dream Vanilla
  BLEND WITH:
  1 tsp. whey protein
  ½ banana

- 1¼ cups Soy Dream Chocolate
  BLEND WITH:
  1½ tsp. whey protein
  ½ tsp. olive oil

- 2 oz. chicken breast (deli)
  1 mango
  3 Ry-Krisp
  2 tsp. almond butter
  PREPARATION: Melt cheese over chicken; spread almond butter on Ry-Krisp

- Metabolize™ Nutri-Bar*

- Metabolize™ Nutri-Shake*

- Smoothie
  BLEND:
  1 cup orange juice
  ½ cup pineapple chunks
  ⅓ banana
  ¾ scoop whey protein
  1½ tsp. olive oil

- 1 apple
  1 fig
  1 peach
  3 oz. Almond Rella mozzarella cheese

LEAN: NUTRITIONAL BREAKDOWN (1,800 CALORIES)		
Breakfast, Lunch, and Dinner (500 calories each)		
Carbohydrate:	300 calories	75 grams
Protein:	100 calories	25 grams
Fat:	100 calories	11 grams
Snack (300 calories)		
Carbohydrate:	180 calories	45 grams
Protein:	60 calories	15 grams
Fat:	60 calories	7 grams

*For sources of Metabolize™ products: *www.metabolize.net* or 1-800-828-3343

MIXED

SNACKS	❖ (CHOOSE 2 PER DAY)

- 2 oz. chicken breast
  1 oz. Rice Slices American cheese
  1 apple
  1 kiwi
  1 tbsp. lite mayonnaise

- ½ cup cottage cheese (2%)
  1 pear
  2 celery stalks
  2½ tsp. cashew butter (spread on celery)

- Metabolize™ Nutri-Bar*

- Metabolize™ Nutri-Shake*

- Smoothie
  BLEND:
  ¾ cup orange juice
  ⅓ cup pineapple chunks
  ⅓ banana
  ¾ scoop whey protein
  1½ tsp. olive oil

- 1⅓ cups low-fat yogurt
  ½ tsp. slivered almonds (or 1½ whole almonds)
  ½ cup pineapple chunks

- 1 tbsp. lite mayonnaise
  1 slice sprouted grain bread
  1 leaf lettuce
  1 slice tomato (chopped)
  2 oz. turkey breast (deli)
  PREPARATION: Spread mayonnaise on bread; add lettuce, tomato, and turkey for open-face sandwich.
  1 macadamia nut
  1 kiwi

*For sources of Metabolize™ products: *www.metabolize.net* or 1-800-828-3343

MIXED: NUTRITIONAL BREAKDOWN (1,800 CALORIES)		
Breakfast (400 calories)		
Carbohydrate:	200 calories	50 grams
Protein:	100 calories	25 grams
Fat:	100 calories	11 grams
Lunch and Dinner (450 calories each)		
Carbohydrate:	225 calories	56 grams
Protein:	112 calories	28 grams
Fat:	112 calories	12 grams
Snack (250 calories x 2)		
Carbohydrate:	125 calories	31 grams
Protein:	62 calories	16 grams
Fat:	62 calories	7 grams

CLEAN

SNACKS

❧ (CHOOSE 2 PER DAY)

- 1¼ cups low-fat yogurt
  1 tsp. slivered almonds (or 3 whole almonds)
  4 black cherries

- 1 hard-boiled egg
  2 hard-boiled egg whites
  1 tbsp. lite mayonnaise
  pepper to taste
  1 slice sprouted grain bread
  PREPARATION: Mix eggs with mayonnaise; add pepper; make open-face sandwich on bread.
  1 peach

- 2¾ oz. turkey
  1 tbsp. lite mayonnaise (spread on turkey)
  1 pear
  1½ macadamia nuts

- Metabolize™ Nutri-Shake*

- Metabolize™ Nutri-Bar*

- ½ cup cottage cheese (2%)
  2 crushed walnut halves
  1 cup pineapple chunks

- 2½ oz. chicken breast
  1 tbsp. mayonnaise
  1 slice sprouted wheat bread
  PREPARATION: Make sandwich using above ingredients.
  1 cup watermelon cubes
  3 almonds

CLEAN: NUTRITIONAL BREAKDOWN (1,800 CALORIES)		
Breakfast (400 calories)		
Carbohydrate:	160 calories	40 grams
Protein:	120 calories	30 grams
Fat:	120 calories	13 grams
Lunch and Dinner (450 calories each)		
Carbohydrate:	180 calories	45 grams
Protein:	135 calories	34 grams
Fat:	135 calories	15 grams
Snack (2 snacks; 250 calories each)		
Carbohydrate:	100 calories	25 grams
Protein:	75 calories	19 grams
Fat:	75 calories	8 grams

*For sources of Metabolize™ products: *www.metabolize.net* or
1-800-828-3343

SUPER-CLEAN

SNACKS	❖ (CHOOSE 3 PER DAY) There are 2 lists of Super-Clean snacks (200-calorie and 150-calorie). Eat one 200-calorie snack between breakfast and lunch. Then have two 150-calorie snacks later in the day (one between lunch and dinner, and one after dinner).

❖ 200-CALORIE SNACKS (AFTER BREAKFAST)
- 2 oz. low-fat cheddar cheese
  ¾ apple
  3 almonds

- ½ cup low-fat cottage cheese (2%)
  1 peach (slice over cottage cheese if desired)
  1 celery stalk
  2 tsp. cashew butter (put on celery)

- Metabolize™ Nutri-Bar*

- Metabolize™ Nutri-Shake*

- 1 cup yogurt
  1½ oz. turkey
  8 black cherries

- 1 hard-boiled egg
  2 hard-boiled egg whites
  7 grapes
  1 Asian pear
  2 cashews

- 2½ oz. turkey
  1 lettuce leaf
  ¼ tomato (diced)
  1 tbsp. lite mayonnaise (spread on turkey; season to taste; add lettuce leaf and tomato, and roll up)

*For sources of Metabolize™ products: *www.metabolize.net* or 1-800-828-3343

½ kiwi

1 guava

3 almonds

- 2 oz. chicken (deli)
  1 slice sprouted wheat bread
  1½ tbsp. mayonnaise
  1 leaf lettuce
  1 slice tomato
  PREPARATION: Prepare sandwich with above ingredients.

❧ 150-CALORIE SNACKS (AFTER LUNCH AND DINNER)

- 1½ oz. low-fat cheddar cheese
  ½ apple
  2 almonds

- ⅓ cup low-fat cottage cheese (2%)
  1 peach (slice over cottage cheese, if desired)
  1 celery stalk
  1 tsp. cashew butter (put on celery)

- Metabolize™ Nutri-Bar*

- Metabolize™ Nutri-Shake*

- ¾ cup yogurt
  1 oz. turkey
  5 black cherries

- 1 hard-boiled egg
  1 hard-boiled egg white
  1 Asian pear

- 2 oz. turkey
  1 lettuce leaf
  ¼ tomato (diced)
  1 tbsp. mayonnaise (spread on turkey; season to taste; add lettuce leaf and tomato, and roll up)
  1 kiwi

*For sources of Metabolize™ products: *www.metabolize.net* or 1-800-828-3343

- 1½ oz. chicken (deli)
  ½ slice sprouted wheat bread
  1 tbsp. lite mayonnaise
  1 leaf lettuce
  1 slice tomato
  2 tsp. raisins
  PREPARATION: Prepare sandwich with above ingredients. Consume raisins on the side.

Super-Clean: Nutritional Breakdown (1,800 calories)		
Breakfast (400 calories)		
Carbohydrate:	140 calories	35 grams
Protein:	140 calories	35 grams
Fat:	120 calories	13 grams
Lunch and Dinner (450 calories each)		
Carbohydrate:	157.5 calories	39 grams
Protein:	157.5 calories	39 grams
Fat:	135 calories	15 grams
Snack (3 snacks total)		
(200-calorie snack; 1 per day)		
Carbohydrate:	70 calories	17.5 grams
Protein:	70 calories	17.5 grams
Fat:	60 calories	7 grams
(150-calorie snacks; 2 per day)		
Carbohydrate:	52.5 calories	13 grams
Protein:	52.5 calories	13 grams
Fat:	45 calories	5 grams

With the food lists and sample menus for your Metabolic Type by your side, and with the dietary suggestions in this chapter as additional guides, it is finally time to begin the *Metabolize* diet. Many people find it helpful to keep a diary of all the food they consume, particularly in the first week or so of making significant changes in their diet. It provides a written record of whether they're making appropriate food choices for their Metabolic Type, and it can point out those areas where they need to improve.

Use the charts that follow to write down your dietary choices on *Metabolize*. There are enough charts for the first three days of this program. I suggest making photocopies of the charts for at least the first week.

I am Metabolic Type (circle one):

Super-Lean

Lean

Mixed

Clean

Super-Clean

My optimal food ratio is:

_____% carbohydrate

_____% fat

_____% protein

DAY 1 ON *METABOLIZE*

Foods I ate today _____
                        (date)

BREAKFAST

CARBOHYDRATES:

Grains _____

Fruits _____

Vegetables _____

PROTEINS:

Meat/Fowl _____

Seafood _____

Dairy _____

FATS:

Nuts/Seeds _____

Oils _____

Other Fats _____

LUNCH

CARBOHYDRATES:

Grains _____

Fruits _____

Vegetables _____

PROTEINS:

Meat/Fowl _____

Seafood _____

Dairy _____

FATS:

Nuts/Seeds _____

Oils _____

Other Fats _____

Dinner

CARBOHYDRATES:

Grains _____

Fruits _____

Vegetables _____

PROTEINS:

Meat/Fowl _____

Seafood _____

Dairy _____

FATS:

Nuts/Seeds _____

Oils _____

Other Fats _____

Additional Meal or Snacks

CARBOHYDRATES:

Grains _____

Fruits _____

Vegetables _____

PROTEINS:

Meat/Fowl _____

Seafood _____

Dairy _____

FATS:

Nuts/Seeds _____

Oils _____

Other Fats _____

After eating my meals today, my general feeling of well-being had the following rating on a 1 to 5 point scale (with 1 representing feeling tired or run-down, and 5 representing feeling great).

1   2   3   4   5   *(circle one)*

Day 2 on *Metabolize*

Foods I ate today _____
(date)

Breakfast
CARBOHYDRATES:

Grains _____

Fruits _____

Vegetables _____

PROTEINS:

Meat/Fowl _____

Seafood _____

Dairy _____

FATS:

Nuts/Seeds _____

Oils _____

Other Fats _____

Lunch
CARBOHYDRATES:

Grains _____

Fruits _____

Vegetables _____

PROTEINS:

Meat/Fowl _____

Seafood _____

Dairy _____

FATS:

Nuts/Seeds _____

Oils _____

Other Fats _____

DINNER

CARBOHYDRATES:

Grains _____

Fruits _____

Vegetables _____

PROTEINS:

Meat/Fowl _____

Seafood _____

Dairy _____

FATS:

Nuts/Seeds _____

Oils _____

Other Fats _____

ADDITIONAL MEAL OR SNACKS

CARBOHYDRATES:

Grains _____

Fruits _____

Vegetables _____

PROTEINS:

Meat/Fowl _____

Seafood _____

Dairy _____

FATS:

Nuts/Seeds _____

Oils _____

Other Fats _____

After eating my meals today, my general feeling of well-being had the following rating on a 1 to 5 point scale (with 1 representing feeling tired or run-down, and 5 representing feeling great).

1   2   3   4   5   *(circle one)*

DAY 3 ON *METABOLIZE*

Foods I ate today _____
(date)

BREAKFAST

CARBOHYDRATES:

Grains _____

Fruits _____

Vegetables _____

PROTEINS:

Meat/Fowl _____

Seafood _____

Dairy _____

FATS:

Nuts/Seeds _____

Oils _____

Other Fats _____

LUNCH

CARBOHYDRATES:

Grains _____

Fruits _____

Vegetables _____

PROTEINS:

Meat/Fowl _____

Seafood _____

Dairy _____

FATS:

Nuts/Seeds _____

Oils _____

Other Fats _____

DINNER

CARBOHYDRATES:

Grains _____

Fruits _____

Vegetables _____

PROTEINS:

Meat/Fowl _____

Seafood _____

Dairy _____

FATS:

Nuts/Seeds _____

Oils _____

Other Fats _____

ADDITIONAL MEAL OR SNACKS

CARBOHYDRATES:

Grains _____

Fruits _____

Vegetables _____

PROTEINS:

Meat/Fowl _____

Seafood _____

Dairy _____

FATS:

Nuts/Seeds _____

Oils _____

Other Fats _____

After eating my meals today, my general feeling of well-being had the following rating on a 1 to 5 point scale (with 1 representing feeling tired or run-down, and 5 representing feeling great).

1   2   3   4   5   *(circle one)*

ENJOYING THE RESULTS

Congratulations on getting started with *Metabolize*. As you adopt this eating plan in the days and weeks ahead, you should begin to experience the first signs of improvement quite rapidly, not only in your weight but also in the way you feel. If you eat in a way supportive of your Metabolic Type, you will notice the results building day after day—and that should motivate you to stick with it.

In the chapters that follow, I'll introduce you to the other elements of the program. Then, in Chapter 13, you'll find the 21-Day Action Plan that ties all of the components, including your eating plan, into a user-friendly package.

This is the start of a new way of thinking about food and total good health. As you nourish your body, you'll also nurture your overall sense of well-being. Now that you've begun, turn the page and discover the rest of *Metabolize*.

Meta-Check

What if you frequently find yourself hungry after adopting this program? What can you do to tame those hunger pangs? Here are some strategies to try:

(Check to make sure you are eating primarily from your Preferred list.

(Monitor your ratios—they matter!

(Do the Wave or even the entire set of the Seven No-Sweat Energy Movements (see Chapter 9). They really work!

(If your Metabolic Type is Lean or Super-Lean, focus on the meats and oils in your Preferred and Sometimes lists. If you are Mixed, Clean, or Super-Clean, concentrate on the meats and oils in your Preferred list only.

(Add an additional snack from your list, or increase your total caloric intake by 200 calories, and see what happens.

7

Supplements:

In Search of That Extra Boost

Everyone's looking for an edge. If you're an elite athlete, you might be seeking a way to slice a fraction of a second off your time in the 100-meter run. If you operate a retail business, you're probably hoping to find the next breakthrough product that can catapult you ahead of the competition. If you're an investor, you could be dreaming that your financial adviser will steer you toward the latest hot stock that can help ensure a comfortable retirement. In short, if there's something that can turn your life around—particularly if it doesn't require too much blood, sweat, and tears—you (and perhaps millions of other people) probably can't wait to get in line.

Not long ago, I heard a story about Arnold Schwarzenegger that dated back to the time when he was pumping iron and growing muscles that seemed to have no limits—long before *The Terminator* was even a figment in a Hollywood screenwriter's imagination. It seems that a fellow competitor at bodybuilding events was so impressed with Schwarzenegger's physique that he asked, "What are you doing differently from the rest of us? Are you taking something? Vitamins? Minerals? Some other type of supplement?"

Schwarzenegger wasn't doing much out of the ordinary—except spending much more time in the weight room than anyone else. His work ethic was phenomenal. But he responded to that question, with tongue firmly in cheek. "Let me tell you what I do," he said, "and you should try it, too." Schwarzenegger advised his colleague, "Consume a sugar cube today. And then for the next thirty days, add an additional sugar cube each day. So tomorrow take two sugar cubes, and then three the following day, and so on. After a month, you'll be taking thirty sugar cubes a day. It will make an incredible difference in your body! Try it and see!"

Amazing! Could anyone possibly buy into the sugar-cube regimen? Well, never underestimate the appeal of a purported magical elixir. Schwarzenegger's fellow bodybuilder couldn't wait for the sugar rush to begin. He hurried to the supermarket, stocked up on sugar cubes, and then began taking them like a Thoroughbred horse in training, just as he had been instructed to do. Each day, the "dose" was a little higher. By day 21, he was absolutely *flying* through the ceiling.

But how did his muscles respond? Well, they didn't exactly cooperate. In fact, he didn't add a single bulge. (What a surprise!) Finally, he figured it out: The joke was on him. He tossed out his package of remaining sugar cubes and returned to lifting weights in earnest.

One of the lessons we can learn from this story is that people everywhere are searching for the next panacea. Maybe that's just human nature. And with health and nutrition in mind, they're often turning to supplements. Americans spend more than $5 billion on supplements each year. They're hoping against hope that these pills have miraculous properties that can cure their ills, make them stronger, shed some pounds, or add years to their life.

When I was in high school, I was desperately trying to become more muscular so I could play football a little better. What was my strategy? Well, the fad of the moment was beef liver tablets—that's right, *beef liver!* It sounded crazy—and it was! But I didn't want to be left on the sidelines by teammates who were popping beef liver like it was Good & Plenty. So I have to admit that I swallowed my share. The beef liver tasted atrocious, so I tried ways to improve the flavor, including mixing it with protein powder in a blender and then drinking it. Ugh! Yes, it looked like a milk shake with chocolate chips in it—but it tasted like mud! Somehow I forced myself to swallow the putrid potion each day, with the unrealistic hope that it would turn me into the next Dick Butkus or Deacon Jones. Of course, that didn't happen. As luck would have it, however, I was moving through an adolescent growth spurt at the time—and was lifting weights at a fanatical pace—and so my weight unexpectedly began to climb quickly, from 165 to 183 pounds, and I felt like I could bench-press the world. But it sure would have been wrong to give all the credit to the beef liver pills.

WHAT ARE VITAMINS ANYWAY?

Looking back, I'm certainly not surprised that beef liver tablets never really caught on for the long term. But you can't say the same about vitamin pills. By far, they're the most popular supplements around. But just what are vitamins?

Vitamins are organic compounds derived from living material (plants, animals) that your body needs only in tiny quantities to maintain good health—that's right, very tiny quantities. While you've probably heard the hype from some supplement gurus that the road to optimal health is paved with *mega*doses of vitamins, there's just not much science to support this "more is better" ideology.

Researchers discovered the first vitamin relatively recently—in 1913, to be exact. It was vitamin A, and when scientists learned that its chemical structure contained an *amine* (a nitrogen-containing compound), they assigned the name *vitamine* (an amine vital to life) to these substances. (The *e* was soon dropped when researchers found that some vitamins are not amines after all because of their varying chemical structures.) Today there are 13 vitamins, which were assigned names beginning with *A* and then generally proceeding down the alphabet in the order in which they were discovered.

So what quantity of vitamins is the right quantity of vitamins? First of all, for optimal health, you need much larger quantities of carbohydrates, fat, and protein than vitamins. Nevertheless, in the proper amounts, vitamins are necessary to keep your body humming full speed ahead. They are crucial for the proper activity of enzymes; without them, important metabolic functions within cells wouldn't occur as they should. Your body requires vitamins for tissue repair, maintaining strong bones and teeth, the manufacture of hormones, the strengthening of the immune system, and the efficient functioning of the heart and nervous system. Although vitamins themselves don't provide energy, they do help convert food into energy.

A recent government study concluded that 90 percent of Americans consume less than the RDA (Recommended Dietary Allowance) of one or more vitamins and minerals each day. That's an alarming statistic, and a clear sign that most people aren't eating balanced meals. Fortunately, if you don't get enough of a particular vitamin in a given day, you can make up for it the next day; your body isn't going to fall to pieces if you eat poorly now and then. But you can get into real trouble if you're not meeting the RDAs meal after meal, week after week, month after month.

If you have a severe vitamin deficiency, it can cause many health-sabotaging diseases and disorders. If you're short of vitamin D, for example, you run the risk of rickets, bone fractures, and muscle spasms. If you're vitamin C–deficient, you could be prone to scurvy, bleeding gums, joint pain, and depression. If vitamin A is scarce in your diet, night blindness and respiratory infections are possible health complications. If you're short of riboflavin, you might develop a skin rash and cracks at the corners of your mouth.

Although vitamins get most of the attention, don't forget about minerals. You're probably already familiar with many of them, such as calcium, sodium, magnesium, and iron, and they're just as important as vitamins. But unlike vitamins, which are organic (carbon-containing) substances, minerals are inorganic (not bound to carbon). But inorganic minerals *do* have a direct effect on our health; a shortage of iron is the most common nutritional deficiency among Americans, causing anemia, fatigue, and a weakening of the immune system.

FOOD OR PILLS?

Although many people seem to buy their supplements by the case, here's the good news: The food on your plate, three meals a day, is your best source of vitamins and minerals.

Fruits and vegetables, for example, contain plenty of vitamins and minerals. They're also rich in antioxidants such as beta-carotene, which can decrease your risk of heart disease and cancer by destroying disease-triggering free radicals in the body. Fruits and vegetables are also excellent sources of fiber, which can further cut your likelihood of developing certain types of cancer (such as colon cancer), while also reducing your cholesterol level.

Here's something else to keep in mind: When you're crunching carrots or other veggies to get your daily infusion of the antioxidant beta-carotene, you'll also be getting plenty of other *carotenoids* (the large group of more than 200 compounds that give plant foods their orange, red, or yellow pigment). Most carotenoids are not as well studied as beta-carotene, but they appear to have plenty of health-promoting properties of their own. For example, research published in the *Journal of the American Medical Association* discovered that certain carotenoids called zeaxanthin and lutein, which are found in spinach, can guard against a common eye disease called macular degeneration; but you're not going to find zeaxanthin and lutein in pill form (at least not yet). So if you're overrelying on supplements, you'll miss out on many dozens of other carotenoids found only in plant foods that can help keep you healthy.

That's why an optimal diet is important—specifically, following the eating program for your Metabolic Type. When you're eating right, you should be able to consume all of the nutrients you need. Just as important, food is relatively free of side effects (which we can't always say about supplements, particularly in large doses).

How Good Is the Food Supply?

There may be a catch, however, when trying to eat optimally. As conscientious as you might be, vitamins and minerals can be lost from food in many ways. In recent years, in fact, many consumers have claimed that the food supply itself as a source of nutrients is suspect. They seem to distrust just about everything that ends up on our plates. For instance, some claim that the soil has been terribly depleted, which in turn reduces the nutritional value of the food that grows in it. I've heard so many conflicting statements regarding this issue that I began doing my own research in hopes of arriving at a credible conclusion.

Well, here's what I've learned: Yes, it's true that during the Great Depression, the soil in the Great Plains was severely damaged by wind, rain, and blinding clouds of dust that whipped through the region. (Hence the area was labeled the Dust Bowl.) But in the years after John Steinbeck's *The Grapes of Wrath* recounted the hardship of Dust Bowl families, the farmers in that region began nurturing their soil back to life. Over the decades, their success in the fields was phenomenal. As a result, *Americans now eat the most nutritious food at any time in our history.*

That point of view was confirmed by many authorities, including Lloyd Shreve, professor emeritus of horticulture at Texas A&M University. He is one of the most respected authorities in his field and has traveled the world helping countries reintroduce native plants that have become scarce or extinct. In a meeting with him not long ago, I posed the following question:

"We've heard so much about how the soil is depleted, and that the nutritional value of the food supply has been terribly weakened. How much of that is true? What's our food supply really like?"

Dr. Shreve offered the following response, which was more than bite-sized in the confidence it conveyed: "The food that's grown in America is *not* depleted by soil erosion. It's that simple."

That was good news, of course. But Dr. Shreve did add this caution: Once food has been harvested, some nutrient depletion could take place before it gets to the dinner table. But, he added, that just isn't his area of expertise.

So I continued my research. Other experts told me that after foods like peas, beans, tomatoes, and spinach are harvested, their chemical structure becomes altered almost immediately. Our ancestors ate food that was grown close by, often on their own land; their meals were typically picked or harvested just hours before they were eaten. But that's no longer the case. Food commonly travels hundreds or thousands of miles from farms to the grocery stores that sell it, and in those two to three days of transport, its taste can become noticeably different. Then, once the food is in your kitchen, cooking kills enzymes and destroys nutrients. Remember, vitamins and minerals are very fragile. And while they're being moved across the country in trucks, being stored in warehouses, and then cooked, they lose some of their nutritional value.

If that's not enough to upset your stomach, we also have to deal with food processing, which also takes its toll. As Dr. David Bresler has written, "By the time most food reaches the supermarket shelves, it has been heated and frozen, beaten and bruised, manipulated and mutilated, and wrapped in a glamorous package that may cost more than the food itself. True, it may look inviting, smell wonderful, and taste delightful. But in the process, so much of its nutritive value has been destroyed that often the food has had to be artificially 'enriched' or 'fortified' in order to restore at least some of its nourishment."

KEEPING THE VITAMINS IN YOUR FOOD

Vitamins and minerals are delicate substances, and they can vanish almost magically from food faster than you can say Harry Houdini. Although supplements can rush to the rescue, the best place to get your nutrients is still from food. So here are a few easily digestible tips to help keep your meals as vitamin-rich as possible:

✔ Whenever possible, eat fresh or frozen vegetables rather than canned. Shop frequently to make sure that your produce is as fresh as possible.

✔ If you do eat some canned foods, store them in a pantry maintained at about 65 degrees. If possible, the pantry should not be close to the stove.

✔ When buying breads and cereals, look for whole-sprouted grains. If they are not available, products fortified with extra vitamins are an acceptable alternative.

✔ When cooking vegetables, steam or stir-fry them. Vegetables retain more nutrients when they're steamed, plus most people find their crispiness appealing.

✔ If you do boil vegetables, use only a small amount of water, and bring it to a boil before adding the vegetables to it. Then remove the veggies from the water as soon as they are a little tender; the more water and the longer the boiling time, the greater the loss of vitamins. Whenever possible, use the vitamin-rich liquid in soups, stews, gravies, and sauces.

✔ Don't soak foods like beans and peas longer than suggested by the package instructions, or you'll risk losing precious vitamins. In the same way, rinsing rice before cooking will remove some of its minerals and B vitamins.

✔ Prepare and serve vegetables in larger rather than smaller sizes. For example, if you cook broccoli spears instead of chopped broccoli, less surface area will be exposed, and thus fewer nutrients will be able to escape. In the same way, carrots cut into large chunks tend to be more vitamin-rich than carrots that are diced.

✔ Serve vegetables as soon as possible after cooking; they'll lose nutrients if they sit too long at room temperature. Keep fresh and cooked foods in the refrigerator and wrapped in plastic or stored in airtight containers.

✔ Bake potatoes in their skin in order to preserve their nutrients.

✔ Keep bread away from the sunlight, which can destroy vitamins like A, D, and riboflavin.

SUPPLEMENTS: DO YOU REALLY NEED THEM?

It's time to make some decisions about supplements. If you follow the eating plan in this book closely, adhering to the diet created for your Metabolic Type, and taking steps like those listed above to ensure that the foods you eat are as vitamin- and mineral-rich as possible, you may not need to take supplements. But frankly, I've found that most people can benefit from at least a modest supplementation program.

Let's face it: Thanks to the fast-paced, hectic lifestyle that most of us lead, we sometimes skip meals and frequently eat on the run. Or we dine in restaurants, where we're served processed food that has been robbed of some of its nutrients. Or we may have allergies that interfere with the metabolism and absorption of certain nutrients in foods. Or we simply find that we just don't eat enough of the right foods to meet our nutritional needs. (For example, to achieve an optimal intake of 1,500 milligrams of calcium per day, you'd have to drink three glasses of milk and eat two eight-ounce servings of yogurt per day, which most people simply don't do.)

So while it's important to stick as closely as possible to the eating plan in this book, why not also take advantage of a relatively low-cost "health insurance policy" that can make certain that you're completely nourished during those times when you can't eat the way you'd like? Supplements also are particularly important for certain groups of people: pregnant or nursing women (who need extra nutrients); individuals who find themselves under frequent and sometimes debilitating stress; and people whose doctors have told them that their digestive system has difficulty absorbing the nutrients they consume (which tends to occur most commonly in older people). Nutritional deficiencies can also occur in smokers (who use up vitamin C more quickly than nonsmokers), heavy drinkers (whose B and C vitamin levels may be depleted), and routine consumers of aspirin (which can interfere with the body's metabolism of folic acid and vitamin C). And by taking a good, well-rounded supplement, you'll be sure to get the proper *combination* of nutrients. (For instance, for the body to properly absorb calcium, it needs to be taken along with some vitamin D—so look for a supplement that contains both.)

AN ALL-PURPOSE MULTIVITAMIN PILL

As part of the *Metabolize* program, I think everyone should consider a daily multivitamin-multimineral tablet. Take it conscientiously, and it can be an important component of your overall health-enhancement program.

When you pop that pill each day, make sure that you take it with some food that contains fat. Eat a little food, take the vitamin-mineral pill, then finish your meal, and the fat in that food will help your body digest the fat-soluble vitamins (specifically, vitamins A, D, E, and K). If you take that pill on an empty stomach, however, much of that pill will not be absorbed by your body. (This is why time-release vitamins don't make sense; if a portion of the nutrient is released when there isn't any fat in your digestive system to help with absorption, much of it will simply go to waste!)

But you don't need to fill your shopping cart to overflowing with bottles of every supplement known to mankind. A simple multivitamin-multimineral tablet is plenty for most people. Of course, if you were to browse through a health food store, you'd find dozens of pills and potions, many that you've probably never heard of, but all of them supported by headline-sized claims—of which you need to be wary. As the saying goes, "If it sounds too good to be true, it probably is."

Some of the available supplements aren't any more nutritious or health-promoting than the bottles in which they're packaged! Yes, my research does show that *some* supplementation *can* support *Metabolize,* but you need to choose wisely. Frankly, taking many of the available supplements doesn't make sense, nor do megadoses of the vitamins and minerals that appear quite valuable in moderate amounts. (Most people need no more than 100 to 150 percent of the RDAs of vitamins and minerals; talk to your doctor before self-prescribing higher doses that can cause toxic side effects.)

In recent years, I've talked to nutritionists, pharmacists, university professors, and everyday people who take supplements, and I've heard every kind of imaginable argument about their benefits and risks. I recall a particularly revealing conversation I had with a professor of pharmacology at a major university. He had been a consultant for a number of supplement companies, and I asked for his opinion on a particular protein drink that he was very familiar with, whose label noted that it contained a mind-boggling 66 ingredients! He smiled and told me, "The first three ingredients are a mixture of proteins, and they *do* have biological value. The other 63 are present in such minute traces that they have no therapeutic significance at all."

"So why were they put in the product at all?" I asked.

"Well, the manufacturer felt it was important to give people what they want. So it includes all the hot substances of the day, such as creatine, chromium picolinate, and ginseng, but in very insignificant amounts. The more ingredients a supplement has, however, the more valuable consumers will think it is—and the more money the company can charge for it."

So when it comes to supplementation, piling on just doesn't make sense. Dr. Linus Pauling was the most prominent of the megadose apostles, claiming that huge amounts of vitamin C could cure the common cold and perhaps more serious ailments. In very high doses, however, many vitamins (most notably vitamin C) are discarded by the body in the urine or perspiration. They're excreted when they pass the saturation point in the body's cells. It's like taking an empty glass, filling it with water, and then keeping the faucet running as water overflows from its edges. That surplus water—just like the excess vitamins you might be taking—will go right down the drain.

But that isn't the whole story. Unlike vitamin C, some vitamins—the so-called fat-soluble ones—*aren't* discarded when they exceed what's needed. They're absorbed in the intestinal tract, and they are stored throughout the body. And that's when trouble may occur. If vitamins accumulate this way, they can become toxic and create chaos with your digestion, absorption, and metabolic balance. In the process, elements of this program could be sabotaged, particularly if these supplements are overstimulating the body's organs as they attempt to process one or more overdominant nutrients.

The reality is that vitamin A is toxic at heavy doses. So are vitamins B_6, D, K, and niacin. And it's not just metabolism that suffers. For example, if you're taking a lot more than 50,000 International Units a day of vitamin A, you could experience possibly permanent effects, such as brain disorders and an enlarged spleen. Doses of vitamin B_6 as low as 200 milligrams per day can cause numbness in the hands and feet and difficulty walking. In short, taking very high amounts of vitamins may do more than deplete your pocketbook; in some cases, it could also be playing Russian roulette with your health.

Whenever you're contemplating taking *any* supplement, ask yourself, "Would I give this to my children?" If the answer is no, either because not enough is known about the supplement—or perhaps because there are clear risks associated with it—then I wouldn't take it myself. My belief is that you can't compromise your future health for something today. So I approach supplements cautiously. When the evidence isn't there, I opt on the side of caution. That has led me to recommend a multivitamin-multimineral pill as part of this program.

CHOOSING THE BEST SUPPLEMENT

There are many multivitamin-multimineral pills available. So which one do you choose? You can shop endlessly, from pharmacies to supermarkets, from health food stores to mail-order houses. Even some department stores sell them. Whenever you shop, here are some guidelines to keep in mind:

First of all, read labels. Choose a multivitamin-multimineral supplement that contains a wide cross section of nutrients. Look for the specific vitamins and minerals in each pill, and their potency. See what you're getting for your dollar, and don't be influenced by glitzy packaging, or bargain-basement prices, or marketing terms like "stress formulas" or "super vitamins." Also, buzzwords like "natural" and "organic" don't necessarily mean that a vitamin is any healthier than its "synthetic" counterpart. Check to make sure that you're getting at least the RDAs (Recommended Dietary Allowances) or DRIs (Dietary Reference Intakes) for each nutrient; these are the *minimum* levels to prevent deficiency-related illnesses; with some vitamins and minerals, higher doses may help promote optimal health.

Next, look for the designation "USP" on the label. The U.S. Pharmacopoeia (USP) is the scientific organization that establishes official standards for drug composition, including quality, purity, and strength. If you see the USP designation on a vitamin label, it means that the contents of the bottle have met the organization's standards. Also check the expiration date; don't purchase any product in which the date has already passed. (As an extra precaution, don't buy vitamins whose expiration date is just a few months away; they could have been packaged years earlier.)

Perhaps the most important factor to keep in mind when choosing a multivitamin-multimineral supplement is to look for one whose nutrients are "food-based." This may not be a term you're familiar with, so let me elaborate a little. As I stated previously, in the best of all worlds you should get all the nutrients you need from food. But because that's not always possible, a single multivitamin-multimineral tablet a day makes sense. And to maximize its benefits, choose those that are not isolated from their food source. Remember, if you swallow the typical vitamin C or vitamin E tablet, all it contains is the vitamin. But that's not the way that nature creates food. You can't go to a farm and pick vitamin C off a tree. You can't harvest vitamin E from the ground. Instead, every vitamin and mineral is part of a food matrix—that is, its molecules are interlaced with protein, fat, carbohydrates, and in some cases bioflavonoids in a very complex structure. That's the way nature intended you to consume them; humans are designed to eat food, not free-form chemicals.

Some supplement manufacturers do their best to deceive you. They'll take a USP vitamin and combine it with bee pollen, or perhaps an herb, and label it a "whole food vitamin." Sure, you might be impressed—but your body knows better. Although the manufacturer has mixed the isolated vitamin with other substances, these probably don't include fat, protein, carbohydrates, or enzymes. It's not the way food occurs in the real world. Vitamins and minerals in nature are part of a food matrix.

A study by doctors Herman Baker and Oscar Frank compared food-based vitamin C with the same vitamin as a USP extract. After two hours in the bloodstream, the absorption of the matrix-based vitamin C was nearly six times greater than the standard USP vitamin C. After eight hours, there was nearly nine times more absorption of the food-matrix vitamin, which rose to more than 18 times after twelve hours. Those are pretty amazing numbers, and they've been confirmed by other investigators.

With data like these, you might think that supplement manufacturers would be scrambling to get their own food-matrix vitamins to the marketplace. But that isn't the case. In fact, you may have to do some searching to find food-matrix vitamins and minerals. Here's the problem: It is a more complicated—and costly—process to manufacture these supplements than traditional vitamin pills. For that reason, these products tend to be more expensive at the retail level.

Yet even though vitamins and minerals blended with a food source may force you to dig a little deeper into your pocketbook, I think you should still consider taking these supplements because of their clear health benefits. And where can you find them? Check at your local health food stores. Look for terms such as "food matrix" or "food based" on the label. If you have difficulty finding these products, turn to appendix B, which provides information about food-matrix supplements that my company, the Biodynamics Institute, makes available through mail order, and that have been especially formulated for each Metabolic Type; or contact the Institute at (877) KEN-BAUM or on the Internet at *www.metabolize.net*.

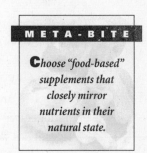

META-BITE

Choose *"food-based"*
*supplements that
closely mirror
nutrients in their
natural state.*

Here's the Bottom Line . . .

We live in a world of fast pace and fast food. So if you occasionally find yourself veering off the dietary program for your Metabolic Type, then a single multivitamin-multimineral pill should be on your own Dean's List of Optimal Nutrition. It can be a wonderful complement to the core of this program and a relatively inexpensive way to compensate for any inappropriate food choices, or for foods that may be nutrient-deficient because they've lost something in shipping, processing, or cooking. But remember that if you're going to take vitamins and minerals in high dosages that exceed recommended levels (more than 100 to 150 percent of the RDAs), I recommend doing so only under the supervision of a doctor. Frankly, if Mother Nature had intended us to take these essential nutrients in extremely high doses, our unprocessed foods would contain much more of them.

Another important caveat: Even the best supplement in the world won't make up for a poor diet or other unhealthy habits. Some people think that vitamin tablets are nothing short of magical, somehow compensating for all kinds of lifestyle shortcomings, such as eating a very high-fat diet or smoking cigarettes. But if you consistently stray from the eating plan for your Metabolic Type, *no* pill will keep you on track for optimal health. If you're consuming a poor diet plus vitamins, it's still a poor diet! One of the basic facts of nutritional life: You won't find good health in a bottle.

CAN VITAMINS REALLY PREVENT CANCER?

Does your doctor roll his or her eyes when you ask whether it makes sense to take vitamins? Many physicians scoff at the mere idea of supplementation—or at least they used to. For many years, the party line of the medical establishment relegated vitamins to the fringes of health care: If you eat a balanced diet, doctors and dietitians said, supplements just aren't necessary. Thanks to some recent research, however, that stubborn viewpoint has softened.

The supplements that are getting the most attention these days are antioxidants—most commonly, vitamins C, E, beta-carotene (a precursor of vitamin A), and selenium. These nutrients neutralize and destroy some of the most potentially dangerous enemies within the body—namely, free radicals. These free radicals are cell-damaging chemical compounds that are a by-product of the natural processes that create energy—much like the harmful gases emitted through the tailpipe of your car that are part of its normal operations. But like rust that attacks metal, these free radicals can bruise and batter your health and well-being—and worse. They can injure DNA, causing cell damage. They can also contribute to serious diseases such as cancer, atherosclerosis, heart attacks, stroke, and cataracts.

But antioxidant supplements can race to the rescue! They defend the body by blocking injury at the cellular level. And the results can be dramatic. Antioxidant research is one of the hottest areas in nutrition these days. For example:

✔ An eight-year-long study by Finnish researchers found that adults with low blood levels of alpha-tocopherol (vitamin E) were 1.5 times more likely to develop cancer than men and women with higher levels.

✔ In a study of 1,300 men and women in the Boston area, those who consumed the greatest amount of beta-carotene had a 75 percent lower likelihood of having a fatal heart attack over a five-year period than those who consumed the least.

✔ Researchers at the National Cancer Institute found that men and women with the highest consumption of dietary vitamin C had a 34 percent reduced chance of developing lung cancer during a 20-year period than those consuming the least amount.

Keep in mind that by following the eating program for your Metabolic Type, your diet will provide your body with an enormous shield of protection from illness. Food should be your primary defender. But a little supplementation like the kind described in this chapter may also be just what the doctor ordered to maximize your overall health and well-being.

8

The Power of Breathing

"Life is in the breath. He who half
breathes, half lives."

PROVERB

How frequently do you think about
your breathing? Probably not very often. Even though you take thousands
of breaths a day, this life-sustaining process almost always occurs unconsciously, much like the beating of your heart.

Nevertheless, breathing is, quite literally, a way of life. Without it,
even for just a short period of time, you wouldn't survive. You can live for
30 days without food and three days without water. But after just six minutes without the nourishing oxygen that breathing provides, you would
be on the brink of death.

Beginning with your very first crying breath at the time of birth, your
body has required oxygen to perform all of its physiological functions.
Breathing oxygenates the blood. It makes possible proper metabolism
and the nurturing of every cell and tissue. In a process called *cellular respiration,* oxygen produces the energy that the body requires. Breathing
also stimulates the body's production of a key molecule that I mentioned
briefly in Chapter 2. Called ATP (adenosine triphosphate), it is present in
every cell. Correct breathing begins the processes by which all of the

proper chemical reactions occur in the body to produce ATP, which keeps the body working efficiently on a cellular level. But when ATP is in short supply, the body feels it. Low levels of ATP can lead to fatigue, lightheadedness, and the buildup of carbon dioxide in the blood.

Something as simple as breathing can have a major influence on your health and well-being. But if you're like most adults, you're probably doing it wrong! Don't let that discouraging thought leave you gasping for air; in the following pages, you'll find out whether you're breathing efficiently and, more importantly, how to use simple health-promoting exercises to breathe as though your life depended on it. (And it does!)

HOW DO YOU BREATHE?

Before we go any further, let's take a moment to analyze your own breathing. Do you breathe up in the chest (a so-called thoracic or chest breather)? Or down in the belly (a diaphragmatic or belly breather)? Do you breathe through your nose? Through your mouth? Or a combination of the two? Are your breaths long or short?

If you're like most people, you probably don't even know how you breathe. Because it's done unconsciously, few people ever think about it. But for the next few minutes, let's change that. Spend some time paying attention to your breathing, without trying to alter it in any way—at least not yet. Just get a sense of your breathing patterns, and what parts of your chest and abdomen are moving as you inhale and exhale.

To make this process easier, here's an exercise you can try:

CHECK YOUR BREATHING

To begin, sit or stand comfortably. Place one hand gently on your belly, positioning the center of your palm over your belly button. Next, rest the other hand on your upper chest, with your fingers just below the collarbone. Now, begin to breathe in the way you normally do. Inhale . . . exhale . . . inhale . . . exhale. As you breathe, watch your hands. Which hand is moving? The hand on your chest? Or the one on your belly? Or both?

As you inhale, if the hand on your chest rises more than the hand on the belly (or if it doesn't move at all), you're a thoracic or chest breather.

Conversely, if the hand on your belly moves the most, you are a belly or diaphragmatic breather.

Most adults are chest breathers—even though diaphragmatic breathing is the healthiest way to move air in and out of your body. If you want to see an example of ideal breathing, watch a baby. He will take deep, rhythmic breaths from the belly that push the diaphragm down with each inhalation, filling up the entire lungs with air, starting with the lowest regions and working upward; then his diaphragm will relax as he exhales. Most of the movement occurs in the baby's belly as it rises and falls effortlessly; look for a bit of a pot belly each time he inhales.

Belly breathing is the natural, instinctive way that all of us once breathed. But somewhere along the way to adulthood, it got lost. Like most adults, you probably breathe high in the chest, which is a constricted way to breathe and leads to short, choppy breaths. As a result, carbon dioxide is more likely to build up in your bloodstream, which can interfere with mental concentration and physical coordination. Nevertheless, you've probably been told that this is the *right* way to breathe—chest out, stomach in—but that just isn't the case.

Later in this chapter, you'll learn how to breathe diaphragmatically by inhaling through the nose and moving the air deep into the lungs. Your belly will "bulge" as you inhale, while the upper chest will remain stationary. This way of breathing is not only good for your overall physical health but will calm you emotionally and help focus your attention.

This way of breathing is called "diaphragmatic" because the diaphragm—the sheath of muscle that separates the chest cavity and the lungs from the abdominal organs—descends farther than it does during chest breathing, making more room for the lungs to expand. When you breathe this way, much more oxygen will reach the lower lobes of the lungs. These lower sections of the lungs have a much greater capacity to absorb oxygen, and as a result, more blood is oxygenated, which in turn facilitates the body's production of ATP. That allows much more efficient movement of waste products (such as carbon dioxide) from the lungs. On the other hand, if you're breathing from your thorax, you use a much smaller portion of your lung capacity; this forces your heart to work harder, in order to ensure that enough oxygenated blood is pumped

META-BITE

By breathing
diaphragmatically,
you can improve your
overall physical and
emotional health.

throughout the body. By breathing shallowly, you also won't expel carbon dioxide from the lungs as efficiently as a diaphragmatic breather does. Thoracic breathing is simply much more taxing on the lungs and other organ systems. So isn't it time to change?

BREATHING AND STRESS

Usually we inhale and exhale about a pint of air per breath. During periods of stress, anger, or excitement, however, as breathing speeds up and becomes shallower, it tends to occur in the uppermost (and least-efficient, in terms of oxygenation) regions of the lungs, and its rhythm becomes irregular.

Stress, of course, is an everyday fact of life. It manifests itself on the freeway when you're going nowhere fast in the midst of a traffic jam. Or when you're arguing with your teenage son over taking out the garbage. Or when you're nervous about an imminent job interview . . . or anxious about a long line at the bank . . . or being berated by your boss (or your publisher) for missing a deadline. When events like these happen, the body's stress response takes over, triggering constricted and choppy breathing that only exacerbates the tension you're already feeling.

The stress response—the so-called "fight or flight" mechanism—is controlled by a part of the brain called the hypothalamus. When faced with a real or imagined "threat," the hypothalamus activates the sympathetic nervous system, preparing the body to either fight off the perceived danger or run from it. As part of this process, which is as old as our most ancient ancestors, a cascade of involuntary physiological events shifts the body into something resembling a state of emergency. Stress chemicals (like adrenaline and noradrenaline) are released, flooding into the bloodstream and speeding up the heart rate, boosting blood pressure, raising blood sugar levels, tensing muscles, and accelerating perspiration. And as I've already pointed out, it also alters our breathing patterns. As respiration becomes choppy, our thought processes may become impaired, leaving us feeling a little less sharp. Food won't be digested and metabolized as efficiently, largely because the body is diverting energy to the muscles. All of our physiological systems, in fact, are put on overload.

When stress becomes chronic—perhaps due to worry over a serious family illness or ongoing financial problems—it can gradually wear down the body, as though you were stepping on the accelerator and the brake of your car simultaneously.

The same stress that often triggers chest breathing can also contribute to many life-disrupting and serious illnesses. Headaches and back pain have been linked to stress. So have high blood pressure, ulcers, asthma, and perhaps cancer. Dr. Herbert Benson of the Harvard Medical School estimates that 60 to 90 percent of all visits to doctors' offices are stress-related.

In her book *Healing Mind, Healthy Woman,* psychologist Alice D. Domar describes an association between shallow breathing, chest pain, and heart disease. She also points to breathing disorders in people experiencing health problems as diverse as fibromyalgia, TMJ, and irritable bowel syndrome. This kind of link, she notes, is not surprising, since "every one of our billions of bodily cells requires oxygen as a source of energy."

CAN STRESS BE GOOD FOR YOU?

If one of your reasons for reading this book has been to learn ways to lose weight, then the following statement may sound encouraging, at least at first glance: *Some people actually lose a few pounds when they're under stress.* But this is certainly not a healthy kind of weight loss. Not only does the digestive system nearly shut down in the presence of stress, but people simply lose their appetite, or even just stop eating. This dramatic decline in caloric intake translates into weight loss. In some cases, however, the reverse is true—that is, people may continue to eat normally during stressful times, but when they do, they're actually more likely to pack on a few extra pounds, thanks to stress-related disruptions in breathing, digestion, and metabolism.

So how should you respond to stress and get healthful breathing back on track? I tell my clients to concentrate on their breathing when their anxiety levels are going through the roof. You should do the same. Consciously bring your breathing from high in the chest to deep in the belly. To begin the process, I often suggest taking just a single deep breath, which in seconds can remarkably calm and comfort you—and actually stop the stress response in its tracks. This slow abdominal breath should include a purposeful and explosive blowing out, not a prolonged sigh that has a "woe is me" feeling to it and can actually create more tension, not less. When done properly, a single deep breath can bring your breathing under control, relax the belly muscles, and normalize the metabolism in every cell in the body. It also can release tension from throughout your body. It is literally a welcome sigh of relief.

Have you noticed what basketball players often do just before shooting a free throw? Many of them pause for a moment and take a single deep breath. Then they breathe comfortably and easily, which relaxes and empowers them before taking the shot. Without those brief moments of relaxation, particularly in a pressure-packed moment of the game, the stress of competition could sabotage their performance.

Perhaps you remember Game 1 of the NBA finals in 1995, in which Orlando Magic guard Nick Anderson went to the free-throw line in the final seconds of regulation, with a chance to win the game for his team. During the season, Anderson had proven his talent as a clutch performer at the free-throw line. Everyone was confident that he would perform this time, too—everyone, that is, except Anderson himself. In this pressurized moment, he seemed unusually tense. His first shot went awry. Then, as he prepared for the second one, you could see the strain in his breathing and almost feel the tension in his body. Sure enough, he missed the second shot as well.

Moments later, Anderson was fouled again and went to the free-throw line for two more shots. Making just one of them would have won the game for the Magic. But Anderson did nothing to try to relax himself. His breathing was choppy, high in his chest—and the shot wasn't even close. By the time he took the ball for the last of those four shots, he didn't have a chance. Almost hyperventilating by this point, Anderson bricked it. Orlando lost the game in overtime, and the Houston Rockets went on to sweep the four-game series. Anderson was so devastated by his performance that he ended up consulting a sports psychologist.

Not long ago, I witnessed a similar scenario while watching a high school basketball game. A number of college scouts attended the game to watch a particular athlete play; this young player knew that he was under the microscope and felt that his future was on the line that night. As the game began, he glanced up at the scouts in the stands—and he froze. One shot after another was a clunker.

A few minutes into the game, the coach sent this frazzled player over to where I was sitting, in hopes that I could get him back into the game. Clearly the young man had been breathing high in the chest, not low in the belly, and it was sabotaging his play. As play continued on the court, I worked with him for a few minutes, helping him breathe deeply, rhythmically, and diaphragmatically. As his breathing normalized, he relaxed, his confidence began to rebound, and he told me he felt ready to return to the game. Once he started playing again, he sunk one basket, then another. He dominated the court. Best of all, in the weeks that followed, he received the college scholarship he had wanted so badly.

The power of proper breathing has been demonstrated in many settings aside from sports. Consider a report by Dr. Aaron Friedell, published in the journal *Minnesota Medicine,* which reviewed a number of studies showing that breathing exercises—specifically, those emphasizing slow, deep respiration—improved "arterial oxygen saturation" and enhanced the health of people diagnosed with heart disease. Dr. Friedell described a case of a patient with severe angina pain, who eased that discomfort simply by changing his breathing. Dr. Friedell taught many other heart patients the proper way to breathe; not only were some able to reduce or even discontinue their heart medicines, but startlingly, their electrocardiograms (EKGs) became normal after using these respiratory techniques. That's the power of breathing!

LEARNING THE RIGHT WAY TO BREATHE

When you have any type of impaired performance or health problem, think about your breathing. This routine process can have an uncommonly strong influence on your well-being.

The importance of breathing has been recognized for centuries. Yogic tradition has viewed breathing as the vehicle for carrying the human spirit and "vital force." The yogis created a science of breathing called *pranayama.* (The Sanskrit root word *prana* means not only "breath" but also "spirit.") They believed that breathing controls the flow of cosmic life force into the body. Many also said that rather than using years to measure the span of a man's life, the number of breaths was a much better yardstick; a longer life, they believed, belongs to those who breathe slowly and deeply.

Today scientists know that breathing can calm the nervous system and promote greater physical health and well-being. But for breathing to become a healing force, it must be done properly—which means breathing diaphragmatically.

When you breathe properly, here's what happens:

✔ The dome-shaped diaphragm (which stretches over the bottom of the lungs) contracts and descends. It presses down softly on the abdominal organs and creates a vacuum that gives the lungs room to expand fully and fill up with air. At the same time, the belly becomes distended.

✔ Then, as you exhale, the diaphragm relaxes. It moves upward in the chest. The lungs contract and propel air from the mouth and nose.

Diaphragmatic breathing fully oxygenates your blood supply and promotes the efficient exchange of oxygen and carbon dioxide.

THE POWER OF BREATH

Now, it's time to try a breathing exercise. It will get you started on a lifetime of diaphragmatic breathing. Remember, this was the way you breathed as a baby; it's time to do it again.

Go into a quiet room and take the phone off the hook. Loosen tight clothing, such as ties and belts. Use the following text as a guide:

> To begin, lie flat on the floor, with a hardcover book beside you; you'll use this book to keep you aware of the movement of your abdomen during this exercise.
>
> Now, place the book on your belly (lower abdomen) below the rib cage. Position it so that its spine faces your chin. The book will help ensure that you're breathing with your abdomen, not your chest.
>
> Next, gently take a breath through your nose.... Inhale slowly and fully.... Feel the air moving deeply into your lungs and abdomen.... Allow your belly to expand without effort, and as it rises, feel how it pushes the book toward the ceiling. At the same time, your diaphragm will move downward....
>
> Then, once you've fully inhaled, begin to exhale through your nose.... Let the air out slowly, about one and a half times slower than you inhaled.... As you gently let go of this wave of air, feel your belly contract.... Watch the book descend into your spine as you expel all of the air in your lungs....

Next, take another breath.... Inhale deeply and gently, and as you do, push the book upward again.... Then exhale slowly, sucking the book down into your spine.... Get in touch with all of the sensations that are present, and enjoy them fully.

Repeat this cycle, again and again. Inhale ... exhale ... inhale ... exhale.... With each slow, rhythmic breath, your belly will rise as you inhale and contract as you exhale.... The key is NOT to expand your lung cavity, but rather to expand your belly cavity....

Continue to breathe deeply and rhythmically ... deeply and rhythmically. Each breath should be natural, flowing, easy, and deep. Eliminate any stops, starts, or jerkiness in the process.

Keep the book rising and falling ... rising and falling.... Get a sense of your diaphragm pushing downward as you inhale, and upward as you exhale.... Inhale ... exhale ...

This is diaphragmatic breathing.... As you breathe, continue to enjoy the sensations.... Don't force it. Let the belly expand and recede ... rhythmically ... gently ...

Welcome to the world of proper breathing.

How did that feel? Practice this deep abdominal breathing technique for about five minutes at a time. Concentrate on moving your diaphragm as you breathe. Feel the tension leave your body with each exhalation.

This way of breathing may feel awkward the first few times you try it. But everyone can learn it. Make it part of your life. With time, you'll conquer years of improper breathing habits and transform the way you feel.

Some of my clients have told me that they've had to consciously work on this new way of breathing in the beginning. But then it became an everyday part of their lives. To speed up this process, here's what I suggest:

For at least the next week, before you get out of bed in the morning, lie on your back and practice diaphragmatic breathing. Place one hand on your upper chest and the other on your lower abdominals. Breathing through your nose, practice the exercise described above. Soften your abdomen, and feel your belly rise and fall, rise and fall. After five minutes, get up and start your day.

Then, before you fall asleep at night, perform the exercise again while lying in bed. With one hand on your upper chest and the other on your abdomen, focus on belly breathing.

Finally, one or more other times in the day—perhaps during your lunch break at work, or even while stopped at a traffic light in your car— try this same exercise whether sitting or standing. Place your hands in the proper positions, and breathe.

Some people become anxious at the mere thought of trying something new. But give it a try. This is a *relaxing,* not an anxiety-producing process. Yes, perfecting the technique will take some practice. But habits can be changed, even one as basic as breathing. After about a week, in fact, this new way of breathing will start to become automatic. It will unconsciously become the way you breathe all of the time. Don't shy away because you're creating a slight pot belly each time you inhale; it's so subtle that no one will notice. In the process, this diaphragmatic breathing will reduce stressful feelings and help balance your body and overall health.

By the way, if you have poor posture, this could interfere with diaphragmatic breathing. So work on sitting and standing up straight, creating more distance between your breastbone and navel, and then breathe deeply. Feel your belly rise and fall. Sense yourself becoming more invigorated with each breath.

Pucker Up and Breathe!

If you're having difficulty getting the hang of belly breathing—particularly if you find yourself doing more gasping than gentle, rhythmic breathing while inhaling— here's a trick that might help:

As you practice this new technique, try inhaling through pursed lips. Pucker your lips as though you were whistling, and then breathe through your mouth. With your lips pursed, you are more likely to inhale slowly and steadily. You'll slow down the process, and allow yourself to focus on moving air through the lips, down your throat, and distending the abdomen. Then exhale through pursed lips at an even slower rate than when you inhaled.

If you'd like, you can also try inhaling not only through pursed lips but also simultaneously through your nose. This combination works well for some people.

A BREATH OF FRESH AIR

Before we wrap up this chapter, I want to teach you an additional breathing exercise. It's one that I use frequently to produce a rapid, split-second feeling of relaxation. It's a perfect antidote to the stresses of everyday life and can have a powerful effect once you've perfected diaphragmatic or belly breathing. Use it to rapidly break any cycle of tension before it soars out of control.

INSTANT RELAXATION

This technique connects your rhythmic breathing to a cue word or "anchor." You can call on this cue word to instantaneously produce a state of relaxation.

❨   *Close your eyes, and think of a place that is very relaxing to you. Perhaps it's a park bench in your neighborhood. Or a favorite location at the beach, a few steps from the ocean. Or a creek that runs beside your cabin in the hills. My own favorite place is the top of a mountain in Yosemite National Park, where I can look out over the valley and quickly feel a sense of peace.*

❨   *Once you have picked a relaxing site, create a vivid image of it in your mind. What exactly do you see? What colors are present? Is there a gentle breeze blowing? Do you hear any sounds (perhaps the lapping of waves on the shore, leaves rustling near a river, birds chirping in the trees)? What can you smell or perhaps taste?*

❨   *Next, select a word that describes this special place. Choose a word that, in a flash, will allow you to recall everything that is extraordinary about this site. It will become a cue to quickly create relaxation throughout your body. Maybe the word is "love" or "relax." There's no right or wrong word; choose one that feels comfortable for you.*

❨   *Now, take the word that you've selected, and in your imagination, place it in your nondominant hand. So if you're right-handed, put it in your left hand (or vice versa). Notice how the word looks in your hand. How large is it? Does it have a color? Is it in block or cursive lettering? Tucking the word into your hand will help it become a "memory cue" that reminds you that relaxation can occur instantaneously.*

❨   *In a moment, I'm going to ask you to take a deep belly breath. You'll hold the breath for about three seconds and exhale rapidly. Then you'll take a second deep belly breath, and this time, you'll make a fist with your nondominant hand, while cradling your special word inside of it. Next, you'll exhale slowly, and as that happens, you'll open your hand. At that moment, your hand will relax completely, and a sense of relaxation will rapidly envelop your entire body.*

Now that you've learned how this exercise works, give it a try:

❲   *Take a deep and rhythmic breath through your nose, and let it flow gently into your lower lungs and abdomen. Allow your belly to fully expand. Enjoy the sensations of oxygen nourishing every fiber of your being. Hold the breath for three seconds. Then exhale forcefully, expelling all the air from your lungs. Then breathe normally for a couple of breaths.*

❲   *Inhale deeply again with a belly breath. As you do, make a fist with your chosen word tucked securely inside of it. Hold your breath for three seconds. Then slowly exhale as you open your fist. As your hand unfolds, allow it to become limp. Feel the tension and stress leave your hand as deep relaxation embraces it. Then instantly sense this same relaxation spreading throughout your entire body, and say your cue or anchor word.*

❲   *Continue to breathe slowly and rhythmically. Experience all the sensations of relaxation, and enjoy them.*

Practice this Instant Relaxation exercise several times over the next week. Each time you use it, making a fist and then opening it, you'll be conditioning your brain and nervous system to send relaxing sensations throughout your body. Then, any time you feel the need to relax, simply make a fist with your nondominant hand, open it, and allow your special word to instantaneously send soothing feelings throughout your body. Your muscles will relax. Your heart rate will slow. With each inhalation and exhalation, your breathing will become calmer. You'll instantly send the "fight or flight" response running for cover.

Most people find this experience a powerful one. After you've mastered it, use it in your day-to-day life, whenever you need a quick infusion of relaxation. Its effects can be felt instantaneously. When you're rushing to the airport to catch a flight, when your baby is crying uncontrollably, when your teenage daughter has made a mess of her bedroom just minutes before guests arrive, when your temper is becoming short with your spouse or coworker, get the instant relief you need.

For example, picture yourself driving on the freeway. Unexpectedly, a car cuts in front of you, forcing you to hit the brakes sharply to avoid a collision. In the immediate moments thereafter, anger may well up inside of you. Your hands might squeeze the steering wheel tightly. Your breathing may become short, choppy, and concentrated in your upper chest. Welcome to road rage!

In a situation like this, before you do anything rash, use the Instant Relaxation technique. As you feel calm in just a split second, tell yourself, "I am fine." At that moment, you might feel like waving cordially at the other driver, rather than using a more combative hand gesture!

Relaxation is just a breath away. Maybe you can't always change the circumstances of your life, but you can *always* manage your breathing, no matter what the situation. As the title of a popular book proclaims, don't sweat the small stuff. Instant Relaxation helps you calm down, put your life circumstances in perspective, and maximize your metabolism and overall health. It can help you become happier and much more at peace with the world.

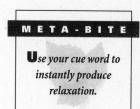

META-BITE

Use your cue word to instantly produce relaxation.

META-CHECK

What if you find yourself becoming anxious, stressed, or lacking in mental clarity? What can you do to turn things around? Here are some strategies to try:

→ Check to make sure that you are eating primarily from your Preferred list.

→ Check your ratios—they matter!

→ Perform the Power of Breath exercise (see page 180) several times a day. Take a few minutes to lie or sit still, and focus on your breathing.

→ Eliminate all wheat products.

→ Eat only those fruits and vegetables that are on your Preferred list.

→ Drink lemon or lime water at least three times a day. Make sure it has plenty of juice and pulp.

→ Add an additional snack to your daily diet, or increase your caloric intake by 200 calories.

9

The Seven No-Sweat Energy Movements

I've been an athlete all of my life. Throughout school, basketball and track were my primary sports, but I've also played football, baseball, and beach volleyball and competed in triathlons. I still surf, rock climb, lift weights, and play a little volleyball. In most of these sports, sweating up a storm is a fact of life.

For the *Metabolize* program, however, don't start stockpiling towels to mop up the perspiration quite yet. Yes, physical activity is a crucial component of this book. But as you'll see, workouts don't have to push you to the brink of collapse to enhance your health.

In this chapter, you'll learn Seven No-Sweat Energy Movements that are the foundation of *Metabolize*'s exercise program. While they'll get your body moving, they won't leave you worn down and burned out— not by a long shot. In fact, most people tell me that with these seven movements, they don't feel like they're exercising at all—which for most of us is the *perfect* kind of physical activity.

Frankly, I don't even think of the Seven No-Sweat Energy Movements as an exercise regimen. I developed them as a way of life, not as the next fitness fad. They are a quick, simple way to integrate whole-body activity into your life, day after painless day. They will improve your coordination, flexibility, and body awareness, while providing an effective outlet for the release of muscular tension. They are perfect for exercise and movement regardless of your Metabolic Type.

THE ORIGINS OF THE MOVEMENTS

Let me give you a little background on how these seven movements evolved. Even though I've always been physically active, I've often forced myself to play through pain. In my early sports activities, many of my coaches promoted the credo "No pain, no gain"—and I was the poster child for playing hurt. I was born with a spinal deformity (the facet joint of my vertebral column is twisted), and I've had to deal with that weakness all of my life. Nevertheless, these physical problems never kept me on the sidelines. I taxed my body to the max and often paid the price with soreness, strains—and a lot worse. I sometimes felt that I was single-handedly keeping the balance sheets of doctors and physical therapists in the black, nursing one back injury after another back to health.

The situation only became worse in more recent years. While training for a triathlon, I took a devastating spill from my bicycle. I slammed into the pavement, and once I stopped bouncing (my friends called me Skip after that), I was carted off to the emergency room with severe back injuries—specifically, a fractured spine and a ruptured disk, both of which required repair work by an orthopedic surgeon. It still hurts to even think about it.

About a year later, with my surgical wounds fully healed, the unthinkable happened. While I was driving not far from my home, an automobile sped through a red light at 50 miles per hour and broadsided my car, propelling it like a bullet across the intersection—and knocking me unconscious. When I awoke in the hospital, the doctors told me that—in addition to suffering a mild concussion—I had ruptured a disk in my back (the same injury I had suffered in the bicycle spill). Before long, I was on my way back to a curtain call in the surgical theater. As Yogi Berra once said, "It was déjà vu all over again."

I spent the next few weeks and months recovering—or at least trying to. The pain persisted and was absolutely agonizing, and it showed no signs of easing. That's when I began a healing sojourn that led me from one treatment guru to another. I tried chiropractic and physical therapy . . . acupuncture and acupressure . . . Rolfing and electrostimulation . . . herbal therapy and self-hypnosis . . . and enough analgesic injections to leave even a pincushion screaming for mercy. Nothing, however, delivered any relief.

I didn't give up. I continued searching for another alternative—one that could not only finally extinguish my back pain for good but also enhance my overall health. I began exploring the possibility of combining the best of Eastern and Western disciplines into a workable system. Over time, I integrated the finest elements of a wide cross section of bodywork and movement into a single fitness program. I drew from the Chinese martial arts such as kung fu and chi kung. I found components of the Feldenkrais system very useful. I adapted elements of American Navy Seal training, U.S. track-and-field conditioning, and traditional flexibility techniques. I combined these elements with state-of-the-art information about human physiology, kinesiology, and biomechanics. Over several years—in consultation with physicians, a chiropractor, a physical therapist, and a certified strength and conditioning coach—I developed, refined, and sequenced the seven easy but powerful movements that I'm about to teach you. Together they can energize the body, revitalize metabolism, and promote optimal health.

DO THEY REALLY WORK?

As you'll see, these movements are simple and easy to use. I've had injuries or other problems involving my back, knee, ankle, ribs, fingers, and thumbs, and I've had no difficulty performing the movements. But despite their simplicity, they can work in powerful ways. Smooth and fluid, they tend to focus on your midsection—the core of the body and the "health center" of your being. These exercises create a balance between body and mind. They also stretch and tone the muscles, promote healthy circulation and blood flow, oxygenate the blood, revitalize sluggish tissue, maintain skin elasticity, and massage the internal organs. They ensure an efficient oxygen exchange that will help properly metabolize the foods you eat, which in turn promotes weight loss. The seven movements also burn calories, which further contributes to the loss of excess pounds. And because they function at your core, they encourage good digestion and absorption as well as metabolism.

Eastern philosophy might tell you that the Seven No-Sweat Energy Movements will stimulate your internal energy source—the Chinese call it *ch'i* —which is one of the keys to unlocking the strength of the entire *Metabolize* program. Chinese medicine is based in large part on the concept of this life energy or *ch'i*. When you are ill, according to this Chinese school of thought, it may be related in some way to an imbalance of *ch'i*. Even if you find this hypothesis difficult to understand, give these seven movements a try. You'll find yourself feeling healthier once these subtle but invigorating bodily movements become a part of your daily routine.

THE SEVEN MOVEMENTS: DOING THEM RIGHT

Before you get started with the Seven No-Sweat Energy Movements (a video is available through *www.metabolize.net* or 1-800-828-3343), let's spend a few moments reviewing some important guidelines. If you follow them closely, you'll increase the effectiveness of these movements:

The Seven Movements
Minimal Pain, Enormous Gain

While the Tin Man in *The Wizard of Oz* may have needed only a squirt of oil to begin moving, your own requirements for jump-starting your internal batteries are a little more complicated. The Seven No-Sweat Energy Movements, however, are actually pretty simple. They are designed for everyone—young and old, healthy and ill. Even if you are coping with ailments such as a stiff back, achy knees, or sore shoulders, these exercises are safe and effective and can provide a healing rejuvenation for the body.

What are the chances of becoming injured performing these seven movements? *Very* slight. After the first time or two that you practice the seven movements, you might feel some soreness (most commonly, in the hamstring muscles). But don't panic. All this means is that you're stretching overly tight muscles, which is all part of the revitalization process.

Even so, keep this caveat in mind: If you experience any *sharp or burning pain,* stop! This kind of discomfort is a signal that something else is going on in your body that needs your attention. Ask your physician for guidance. As a matter of fact, it's best to consult with your physician before beginning any dietary or exercise program.

✔ Perform the movements in the order in which they are presented below, from 1 through 7. They are sequenced in a way so that each builds upon the previous one(s). Do all seven, one after the other, and they'll have a much more powerful, synergistic effect.

✔ Perform all the movements slowly and smoothly. There's no rush; this isn't a competition. As you move through them, avoid jerky or sudden movements. Do not stretch your muscle fibers to the point of triggering an injury (such as a muscle tear). Keep the movements fluid. Stay relaxed.

✔ Breathe in a natural, controlled manner during these movements. That means calmly and rhythmically. Allow your breathing to merge gently with the movements themselves in a harmonious dance. Before you begin each movement, you might choose to take one or more deep breaths to help relax your body and mind; but once you start the movement itself, simply breathe slowly and easily. Avoid explosive exhalations. Don't hold your breath; this will tend only to increase your bodily tension.

Here's a tip that some people find helpful: Purse your lips and breathe lightly through them (and, if you choose, breathe simultaneously through your nose). This will force you to breathe more slowly than you might otherwise do.

✔ Be aware that some of the movements may feel awkward the first time or two you try them. Be patient. Your body needs to become familiar with them. After a few days, they'll become as comfortable as an easy chair.

✔ Pause briefly between movements, just enough to slow your breathing and prepare yourself to proceed smoothly and fluidly to the next movement.

✔ No special attire is needed for these movements. You can perform them in just about any clothes, including a business suit during your lunch break at work. Of course, you should have freedom of movement, so if you're wearing a belt, loosen it. Remove jewelry that might be distracting. Change into comfortable shoes, or remove your shoes completely.

I recommend that you perform the No-Sweat Energy Movements twice a day. They don't take long—just seven to ten minutes for all of them, or only about a minute per movement. I do them first thing in the morning and find that they energize and center me before the activities of the day begin. Then I repeat them in the evening, at least an hour before bedtime; this late-in-the-day session helps remove fatigue and tension from the body; by the time I finally crawl under the covers for the night, I sleep like a baby.

Feel free to choose the best time of day for your own use of these movements. Turn to them whenever you're weary or worn down, or perhaps when you're tempted to eat although you know you really shouldn't. (These movements can quiet hunger pangs, so they're a wonderful alternative to coffee and doughnuts during your midmorning break at work.) If time is at a premium and you just can't squeeze in all seven movements, concentrate on Movement 3—the Wave—which is the most effective "appetite suppressant" of them all; you can even do a version of the Wave while sitting at your desk at work.

Here's my promise: *Everyone* who performs these seven, high-octane movements will feel better afterward. Sure, at first glance they may not seem as appealing as sitting on the sidelines with the TV remote control in one hand and a dish of Ben & Jerry's in the other. But people have told me that they feel a genuine sense of well-being doing the seven movements, as well as a psychological boost knowing that they are actively doing something to improve their health. These simple movements even appear to stimulate the pituitary gland to release a natural opiatelike chemical called endorphin, which produces feelings of contentment in most people and even euphoria in some, while also reducing anxiety, stress, and even physical pain. Ideally, avoid watching television or listening to music while performing the movements; but the important thing is just to do them, so it's better to go through them in front of the TV than not to do them at all.

Here's the bottom line: I predict that you'll become "hooked" on the Seven No-Sweat Energy Movements. Most of my clients have made them as much a part of their lives as breathing and eating.

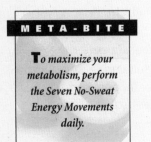

META-BITE

To maximize your metabolism, perform the Seven No-Sweat Energy Movements daily.

THE SEVEN ENERGY MOVEMENTS—PLUS ONE!

It's time to practice the Seven No-Sweat Energy Movements. Use the accompanying illustrations to guide you along.

The first step is to assume a position called the Gunfighter Stance. It is a relaxed posture, free of stress on your joints, that allows your muscles to let go and your breathing to become calm. Let's try it:

THE GUNFIGHTER STANCE

1. To begin, stand with your feet parallel to one another and a comfortable width apart. Distribute your weight evenly on the soles of your feet; avoid leaning too far forward, or back on your heels. Get a sense of how your feet feel when they are balanced on the floor.

2. Assume an erect posture. Avoid bending your spine or arching your back. Keep your spine and neck straight as though there were a vertical pole extending from the tip of your tailbone to the top of your head. Your eyes should be looking forward. Tuck your chin in slightly. Raise your pelvis by pushing the lower part a little forward, and relax your belly.

GUNFIGHTER STANCE:
Posture for Relaxation and Focus

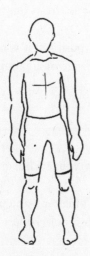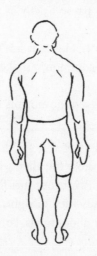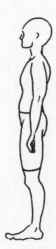

3. Close your eyes, and notice how your body feels. Sense each vertebra resting right where it belongs. Feel your facial muscles relax, and allow your jaw to drop a little, with your mouth slightly open. Do not lift your chin.

4. Next, pay attention to your shoulders. Raise them upward toward your ears, and then round them and allow them to drop down. Let your shoulder blades pull apart a little, and notice a slight space being created in your armpits. Then rotate your arms inward a bit so the inner fold of your elbows is toward your sides. Feel your arms relax and hang loosely as your hands rest slightly forward.

5. Now, concentrate on your lower body. Move your left leg a little to the side so your feet are slightly more than a shoulder-width apart. Bend your knees a little, and check that your toes are pointed forward. Become aware of how comfortable the area between your hips and your pelvis is becoming.

6. Focus on your breathing. Notice how your whole body is calm and centered. Enjoy the sensations of relaxation.

The Gunfighter Stance is the basic posture that you'll use for relaxation and focus. (If you have a bad back, this is a comfortable stance when you need to be on your feet for a long time.) It is also the starting posture you'll assume before beginning the first of the Seven No-Sweat Energy Movements. It can be used as a neutral posture between movements as well—a way to pause briefly as you proceed from one movement to the next.

Because the Gunfighter Stance is an "anchor" position, it is important to get it right. Some common mistakes to be aware of are illustrated on page 195.

Now, let's learn the Seven Movements themselves:

1—FOCUS MOVEMENT

1. Stand with your feet close together, with two to four inches of space between your ankles. Point your toes forward.

2. Take one of your hands—left or right, it doesn't matter—and place it lightly on your lower abdominals. Your thumb should be just below your belly button.

INCORRECT GUNFIGHTER STANCE

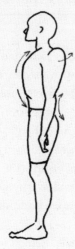

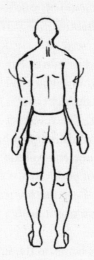

ERROR 1:
shoulders back
chest lifted
belly taut
back arched

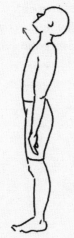

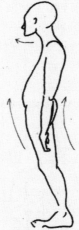

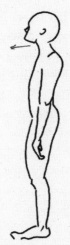

ERROR 2:
chin lifted

ERROR 3:
head forward
spine bent

ERROR 4:
chin slightly forward

3. Place the other hand on the small of your back, above your rear. Your knuckles should be touching your back. Don't apply pressure; let the hand rest lightly.

4. Keep your head erect. Tuck your chin slightly.

5. Now, begin to move your waist in small circles as though you were twirling an imaginary hula hoop around your waist, starting with a motion to the right that is very subtle, perhaps two to three inches of movement. The center of your body—your energy source between your two hands—should be the focus of this movement.

6. After making ten revolutions, stop momentarily, and then change the direction of your circular motion. This time, begin with movement to the left. Keep the motion subtle. Enjoy this slow, rhythmic movement as you continue in a circular pattern for ten additional revolutions.

7. Drop your hands to the side. Inhale and exhale. Return to the Gunfighter Stance, and prepare for Movement 2.

If you are having difficulty performing the Focus Movement, concentrate on keeping the motion slow, controlled, and rhythmic. As you become more proficient at this movement, you'll experience the subtle sensations of generating energy.

MOVEMENT 1—FOCUS MOVEMENT

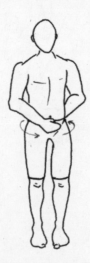

2—TOUCH THE SUN

1. Stand with your feet close together, with about two to four inches between them. Point your toes forward.

2. Interlock the fingers of your hands, and with your hands at about waist level, your palms should face the floor. Then, in a wide circular motion, raise your hands up and above your head. Stretch them high, reaching skyward toward the sun, as though you were trying to lift your upper body away from your rib cage and waist. Hold this position for five to ten seconds, continuing to breathe normally, rhythmically, and smoothly.

3. Release your clasped fingers, but keep them lightly touching once again. Then, in an arcing motion, bring your hands back to waist level.

4. Now, repeat step 2. Interlock your fingers, with the palms facing the floor. Then, in a wide circular motion, raise your hands and arms over your head, and reach toward the sun.

5. As you stretch your arms overhead, twist your torso to the right very slowly, just to the point where you feel a little tension. Then return to the center position, still stretching your arms high overhead. Next, turn your torso to the left very slowly. Then return to the center.

6. Repeat step 5. With your arms overhead, twist your torso to the right, back to the center, then to the left, and finally returning to the center. Repeat these motions one more time: to the right . . . center . . . left . . . center.

7. Release your fingers, and in an arcing motion, bring your hands and arms down to waist level. Breathe.

8. Now, clasp your hands together again, and raise them overhead, reaching once again for the sun. This time, with your fingers still interlocked, lean your body toward the right, slowly, bending and stretching sideways at the waist while keeping your hands above you. After about three seconds, return to the upright position, and then lean and stretch toward the left, slowly. Three seconds later, go back to the center, and then release your fingers. In an arcing motion, lower your arms to waist level.

MOVEMENT 2: TOUCH THE SUN

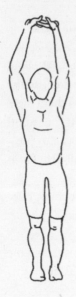 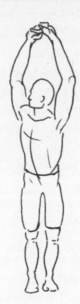 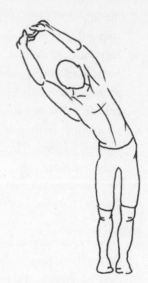

9. Repeat step 8 two more times, raising your interlocked fingers over-head, and then stretching to the right and then the left. Once you've returned your hands to waist level for the last time, relax.

If you become tired during the Touch the Sun movement, particu-larly as you're learning it, it's okay to stop, release your fingers, and relax momentarily. Then continue the motion.

3—THE WAVE

1. Assume the Gunfighter Stance.
2. Place one hand lightly on your abdomen, positioning the thumb just below your breastbone. Rest your other hand on your stomach, slightly below the little finger of the top hand.
3. Inhale, and as you do, feel your belly expanding and your diaphragm contracting. It will look as though your stomach is pushing your lower hand outward. Then exhale, and as your belly retracts, your di-aphragm will push your upper hand out. It's an alternating wavelike

motion. Your stomach extends, your diaphragm contracts; your stomach contracts, your diaphragm extends.

4. Now, with your hands in the same position, rotate your upper body to the right, do the wavelike motion three times, and then return to the center. Next, turn your upper body to the left, and then return to the center. Don't strain during these movements.

5. Repeat the rotations to the right and the left (in step 4) four more times, and return to the center.

The Wave works on the energy center of the body. It relaxes your midsection in particular—massaging the intestines, the stomach, the liver, the kidneys, and other organs. It also loosens up the ligaments and tendons in the region of the spine.

4—HULA HOOP

1. Assume the Gunfighter Stance.

2. Position your feet about a hip-width apart, with your toes directed forward. Place one hand lightly on your belly and the other hand on the small of your lower back.

3. Focus on your midsection, and using your abdominals, begin rotating your waist in a circular motion, moving first to the right. This

MOVEMENT 3: THE WAVE

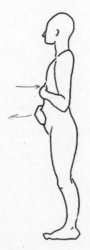 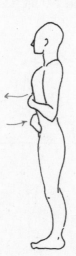 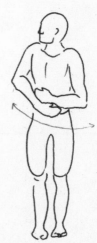

motion is similar to the Focus Movement but in larger circles—about four to six inches of motion. The movement may remind you of the one you used when playing with a hula hoop as a child. As you move to the right, notice how your right hip points slightly to the right. Then, as you make a complete revolution, and come around to the left side, notice that your left hip points slightly to the left.

4. Make ten complete circles while keeping your breathing relaxed and controlled. Your movement should be rhythmic and easy. Do not rock from side to side.

5. After ten revolutions, change the direction of the circles, moving to your left side as you begin each new revolution.

Although Hula Hoop is similar to the Focus Movement, it is a little more intensive. By concentrating on your midsection, you'll improve the energy flow in this part of your body, keeping the internal organs functioning efficiently and helping your body absorb nutrients.

5—PARALLEL ARM MOVEMENT

1. Stand with your feet and ankles almost together although not quite touching. Keep your head erect, with your chin slightly tucked. Breathe deeply and rhythmically.

MOVEMENT 4: HULA HOOP

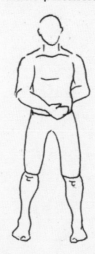

2. Raise your right arm in front of you, extending it outward at shoulder level, with your palm facing down. At the same time, raise your left arm behind you, extending it at shoulder height, with the palm down.

3. Now, swing your left arm forward while moving your right arm back, essentially switching their positions. Allow your pelvis and hips to gently turn as your arms swing.

4. Continue changing the positions of your arms, forward and back. Get into a rhythm. Keep the motion smooth. Complete ten full repetitions.

Before going on to Movement 6, take a short break—a Neck Roll that will release any tension that may still be lingering at this point. Here is how to proceed:

NECK ROLL: THE PAUSE THAT REFRESHES

1. While standing, drop your head forward very slowly and gently. Your chin should almost touch your chest. Feel the gentle stretch in your neck. Hold this position for two to three seconds, and then raise your head upright and relax.

MOVEMENT 5: PARALLEL ARM MOVEMENT

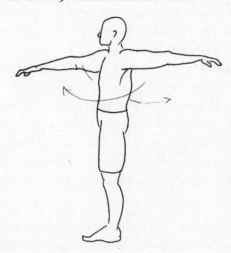

2. Slowly tilt your head to the right, moving your right ear next to your right shoulder. Hold for two to three seconds, and then return to the upright position. Relax.

3. Gently tilt your head to the left, moving your left ear next to your left shoulder. Hold for two to three seconds, and then return to the upright position. Relax.

4. Slowly tilt your head back and look toward the sky. After two to three seconds, return to the upright position. Relax.

Now, let's proceed with the remaining No-Sweat Energy Movements.

6—SIDE STRETCH

1. Stand up straight, with your feet together and your arms at your sides.

2. Take a side step with your left foot, thus spreading your feet so that they're a little more than a shoulder-width apart. Point your toes forward.

3. Place your right hand on your right hip. Lift your left arm, and lengthen your torso as you stretch the arm upward, straight above your head, with your fingers pointing toward the sky. Your left palm should face inward.

4. Now, bend your right knee, and shift your body weight onto your right leg. Lean to the right, and as you do, stretch your left arm up and over your head, as far as the arm can go without straining. Feel the stretch, and hold this posture for three seconds. Then return to the starting position in step 2.

5. Next, place your left hand on your left hip. Lift your right arm and stretch it upward, straight above your head, with your fingers pointing toward the sky. Keep your right arm facing inward.

6. Bend your left knee, shifting your body weight onto your left leg. Lean to the left, and as you do, stretch your right arm up and over your head, as far as the arm can go without straining. Feel the stretch, and hold this position for three seconds. Then return to the starting position.

The final exercise will tie together all seven of the No-Sweat Energy Movements. While building strength and flexibility in the waist and

Movement 6: Side Sretch

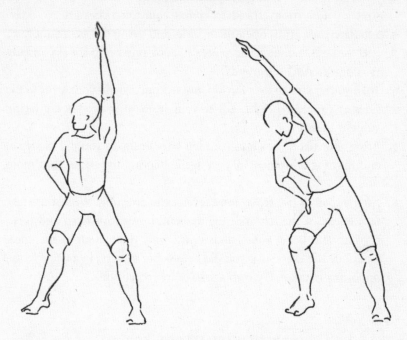

lower back, it will leave you with energized feelings and a sense of well-being.

7—AIN'T LIFE GRAND

1. Assume the Gunfighter Stance.
2. Take a step forward with your left foot so that it is about six inches ahead of your right foot. Bend the left knee slightly; the toes of your left foot may point a little to the left.
2. Bend your head and torso forward as you slide both of your hands down your left thigh to the knee. Do this in a very slow, controlled manner. Your right leg can bend slightly. When you begin to feel a stretch, stop and hold this position for two to three seconds.
3. Begin to rise, while turning your waist toward the left and starting to move in a circular motion. Keep your hands together and raise them overhead. Continue to move into an upright position, with your arms above you.

4. Once in a fully vertical position, lift your chin, look upward, and stretch your arms overhead, extending your torso skyward.
5. Separate your arms, open them wide, and turn your palms upward. Feel the stretch. Enjoy a deep breath. Look up toward the sky and say to yourself, "Ain't life grand!"
6. Turn your palms so they face downward, and extend your arms to the sides at shoulder height. Lower your head so your eyes are facing straight ahead.
7. Bring your hands down to your left knee again, as you did in step 2, and start the movement all over again. Repeat this process four more times.
8. After a total of five repetitions, reverse the direction. With your right foot ahead of the left and slightly bent, move your head and torso forward and bring your hands down your right thigh to the knee. Continue the exercise as you did before, but moving in a circle in the opposite direction. Perform a total of five repetitions.

SHOULD YOU SWEAT, TOO?

On late-night television, it's hard to escape the infomercials for every imaginable type of exercise equipment. If you believe the hype, one piece of apparatus can pump up your biceps, while another can shrink your buns. Still another promises to reduce your belt size, while another gives you more shapely legs. But although many millions of dollars of fitness equipment are purchased each year, most of the apparatus ends up in the same place—under beds or in closets, collecting dust.

The problem is that exercise needs to be highly individualized. Just like dieting, one size doesn't necessarily fit all. What works for Suzanne Somers or Christie Brinkley on those infomercials may bore you to tears, particularly after its novelty wears off. That's why there's always a new product on the market that pledges to finally deliver you to the Promised Land of Flawless Physiques. (By the way, those celebrities probably have personal trainers to help them achieve their model-thin looks!)

When I created the Seven No-Sweat Movements and fine-tuned them, one of my overriding motivations was to develop a program that people could really live with, day after day. As you've seen, these move-

MOVEMENT 7: AIN'T LIFE GRAND

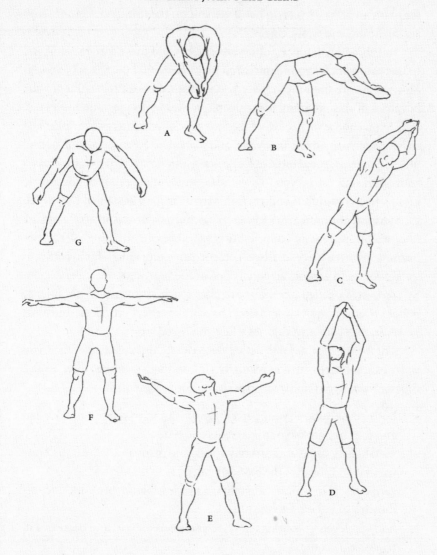

ments take just minutes to perform, they are pain-free, and they are so invigorating and even enjoyable that most people are able to keep their commitment to turn them into a permanent part of their lives. Regardless of your Metabolic Type, the Seven No-Sweat Energy Movements can significantly contribute to reaching and maintaining your health goals, from losing weight to reducing stress to preventing chronic illnesses.

Concentrate on these seven movements, especially if you've been inactive for many months or years. They'll get you on the fast track toward long-lasting health and well-being.

But should you do any other exercise beyond these core movements? In this program, it's your choice. You may decide that the Seven No-Sweat Movements are the only activity you want to do. And that's fine for the purposes of this program. Some people, however, decide to do more.

If you choose to go beyond the Seven No-Sweat Energy Movements, I suggest that you add both *aerobic* and *anaerobic* exercise to your overall fitness program. An aerobic exercise is any physical activity that increases your heart rate, causes you to breathe deeply, and uses your major muscle groups in a continuous and rhythmic manner for a sustained period (20 to 30 minutes or more). Aerobic exercises burn calories and accelerate the rate of thermogenesis (calorie-burning). Rises in this rate of calorie-burning of even two to three percent can contribute significantly to weight loss, and aerobic activity is one of the best ways of accelerating it. By contrast, so-called *anaerboic* exercises (such as push-ups) are intense but are over very quickly and don't have much effect on calorie-burning; however, they can burn calories when you're sedentary.

The benefits of aerobic activity are clearly documented. When you walk, run, swim, or bicycle regularly (for 20 to 30 minutes, three to five times a week), your body will experience improvements in:

✔ body composition (your percentage of lean mass relative to body fat, and the strength of your ligaments and tendons)
✔ metabolism of fat and carbohydrates (the manner in which the body uses fat and sugar in the bloodstream)
✔ cardiovascular fitness (including lowering blood pressure and increasing circulation to the heart)
✔ body fat levels (elevations in HDL cholesterol levels, and decreases in triglyceride counts)
✔ bone strength

If you decide to add some aerobic activity to your life, I'm convinced that walking is the best choice for most people. Because I was a trained athlete, I never thought I'd be content getting my exercise by walking. But in the wake of a number of injuries, I walk more than run these days. For-

Aerobic Activities	Anaerobic Activities
Walking at a moderate to vigorous pace	Sit-ups, push-ups, pull-ups
Running, jogging	Weight lifting
Hiking	Sprinting short distances
Swimming	Housework
Bicycling (outdoor, stationary)	Gardening
Rowing (outdoor, stationary)	Metabolize Stretch & Flex*
Cross-country skiing	
Stair climbing	
Jumping rope	
Step or dance-exercise aerobics	*Call 1-800-828-3343 for ordering
Metabolize Stretch & Flex*	information.

tunately, nearly everyone can walk. Even if you haven't exercised in years, and even if you're significantly overweight, you can still walk (although you should have a medical checkup first if you have a history of health problems such as heart disease, high blood pressure, or lung disease). Unlike running, walking doesn't involve violent pounding of your joints, and thus it carries a very low risk of injury. Its cardiovascular benefits are well documented. So is its ability to burn calories (at a pace of three to four miles per hour, walking zaps about 300 to 400 calories per hour).

Aerobic exercise doesn't require investing in special equipment besides a good pair of walking shoes or high-quality running shoes. Even on cold or rainy days, there are no excuses; you can walk indoors at a local shopping mall. Sure, you've been walking all your life, but I want you to really concentrate on keeping your posture erect, swinging your arms freely at your sides, and maintaining a rapid but nevertheless comfortable pace.

Buy a pair of walking shoes that provide good support. They should be lightweight and padded at the heel and tongue. Make sure they bend easily across the ball of your foot and have a cushioned, uplifted sole and good arch support. Wear thick, absorbent socks, too.

Remember, you don't have to climb Mount Everest to get the benefits of exercise; stepping out through your own neighborhood can make you feel great. If you haven't exercised in a while, be content with starting out by walking just a short distance—perhaps only a city block or two. Then increase your activity level a little each day. Just get moving; that's the most important thing. Don't worry about monitoring your heart rate. A good rule of thumb is the following: While walking, you should be able to talk but not sing. If you can sing, you're not moving fast enough, so pick up the pace. If you can't talk, you need to slow down.

If your goal is to lose weight, think about trying to burn about 250 calories a day through exercise (about 40 minutes of walking at a three-miles-per-hour pace), and then also reduce the amount of calories in your diet by about 250. That 500-calories-a-day decrease will translate into the loss of one pound per week.

For personalized training information, see *www.metabolize.net* or call 1-800-828-3343.

What About Strength Training?

If you're striving for total fitness, then you should consider incorporating strength training into your life. This means working your muscles against resistance to improve their strength and tone. In the process, you'll increase your bone density and thus reduce your risk of osteoporosis, while minimizing your chances of developing backaches and other injuries. Even older people can benefit from strength training; it can extend by years their ability to carry out the tasks of everyday living with less effort.

No, this doesn't mean spending many hours each week pumping iron in the gym at the neighborhood Y. Just 10 to 15 minutes, two to three times a week, can make a big difference, and you can use items around your home as "props." Try doing a few arm exercises with one-pound food cans or quart-sized plastic bottles (filled with water or sand). Or invest in inexpensive dumbbells or customized exercise devices for your body size and strength like Metabolize™ Stretch & Flex (developed by Steve Uchytil of the Biodynamics Institute). Always use a weight you can lift without straining. Perform 8 to 12 repetitions of each exercise, exhaling during the exertion portion of the movement. Once you can do 12 repetitions effortlessly, increase the resistance by 5 to 10 percent.

One other note: When you're trying to lose weight, strength training can be particularly important. You want to lose body fat, not muscle mass, and strength exercises will help you in that effort. Muscles are metabolically active and burn calories even while you're at rest. So if you protect your muscle mass, you'll increase the number of calories you burn.

10

Attitudes for Action

Where their health and well-being
are concerned, many people behave like ships without captains. They
drift aimlessly in an ocean of negativity, dropping anchor briefly at one
doctor's office or another, or upon one diet program or another, hoping
for a magical answer to what ails them. Whether they're seeking to get the
upper hand on a chronic illness, become more energetic, or lose excess
weight, they often believe, even before they start, that any effort they
make will ultimately be futile. Even if they learn what they really need to
do to navigate their way to good health, they have trouble taking control,
knowing that their previous attempts have been unsuccessful.

Sound familiar? If your own weight-loss efforts have failed as you've
moved from one diet to another, or if your back pain stubbornly persists
despite frequent visits to a lengthy list of doctors, it's not surprising that
you're feeling frustrated. *Metabolize* is the one program that many people
have been able to stay with for the long term. But in order for *Metabolize*
to be effective, you need to foster and strengthen a positive attitude. You
must believe that you *can* reach all of your health goals.

STAYING MOTIVATED

Most of my clients tell me that once they understand Metabolic Typing, and begin to see some results, they often feel very motivated and begin to anticipate achieving what I have promised—improved overall health, greater energy levels, and weight loss.

Nevertheless, here's a sobering statistic: Research shows that motivation lasts for an average of only about 17 days. That's right, just 17 days. With that in mind, no wonder you may have started diets in the past, only to give up on them after several days or weeks. Change is hard. As Mark Twain said, "Habits are habits. You can't throw them out the window. You have to coax them downstairs one step at a time."

Toward that end, maintaining a positive attitude is crucial. You need to prepare your mind for success. If you approach this program with positive expectations and a strong commitment to stay motivated and stick with it, you *will* succeed. That means making a concerted effort to set aside self-sabotaging thoughts that all of us have from time to time. For example, how often have statements like these run through your head when you've tried other programs?

✔ "Diets have never worked for me before. I guess I'm just not a person who can lose weight successfully."

✔ "I'm sick of feeling deprived on diets."

✔ "I have to go to a lot of business lunches, and it's hard to stick to a program when I'm eating out so much."

✔ "Whenever I've tried to exercise in the past, it's been torture. I always quit after a few days."

✔ "I'm feeling so run-down! How am I supposed to work out?"

✔ "What's the use? I just don't have any willpower. No wonder I'm so overweight."

✔ "There's too much stress in my life to concentrate on getting my physical health in order."

✔ "This diet just doesn't make sense. I'm absolutely sick of eating rice cakes!"

Metabolize is different. My clients tell me that this program makes it much easier to overcome the excuses that they've used in the past. Although *Metabolize* is an eating plan, it is *not* a diet in the traditional sense. It is certainly not like the kinds of diets you've tried in the past—and that's good. After all, the way most Americans eat—whether or not they're trying to lose weight—contributes to the development of heart disease, cancer, and diabetes. In short, "one diet fits all" plans can kill you! In the same way, while *Metabolize* includes physical activity, it is nothing like the exhausting kind of exercise that you may be familiar with—but it is amazingly effective.

So if you have memories of disappointments with previous diets, set them aside. If you've failed when trying to adopt an exercise program in the past, put that out of your mind. For your well-being, today and in the future, you need to dedicate yourself to this program and not allow the snowdrifts of negative experiences to bury your spirit and extinguish your dreams. You *can* set aside your harmful health habits, but you need to dump the negativity if you are to achieve good health and longevity.

DO YOU HAVE THE RIGHT ATTITUDE?

Your attitude counts. Because a positive "can do" outlook is crucial to staying on track with *Metabolize,* you need to nurture thoughts like "In this program, I get to choose healthy foods, feel my energy level rise, and improve the way my body looks. I'm going to enjoy the process of becoming healthier."

I frequently work with athletes at all skill levels, helping them excel to their fullest potential. A message that I always give them is especially applicable here:

"The more you expect from a situation,
the more you will achieve."

Think about that statement for a moment. Just like the tennis player who fully expects to rebound in the final set to win the match, your own great expectations can produce magnificent results. In the same way, modest expectations tend to deliver only mediocre results. When your health is concerned, you'll experience much more improvement if you're reaching for lofty goals than if you expect to just tread water. Research shows that when cancer patients, for example, are actively *determined* to beat their disease, their chances of conquering cancer are much higher than if they just passively *hope* to survive.

When you consider the possibilities and *really* believe that genuine health enhancement is within reach, then your enthusiasm for this program will soar. Turn yourself over to transforming your life and your health. Remind yourself that you deserve everything that this program can deliver, and really believe it. There is nothing as powerful as a made-up mind.

For maximum results, allow your positive attitude to "infiltrate" every aspect of your life. Here's one way you can start off every day the right way, and avoid "waking up on the wrong side of the bed":

POSITIVE WAKE-UP CALL

Before you get out of bed in the morning, think of some of the things in your life that you're grateful for. Perhaps you're thankful for your spouse . . . for the good health of your family . . . for having a secure job.

This is a simple process. But it will help awaken positive feelings within you (even though it doesn't mean discounting any personal problems you also might have). Let's face it: You're almost always going to be dealing with one problem or another in life—whether it's the stack of bills on your desk or your child's difficulties at school. But if you start the day with positive thinking, you'll equip yourself with the mindset not only to better handle those problems but also to integrate the healing elements of this program into your life.

WHAT ARE YOUR PRIORITIES?

Let's pause a moment and start to examine your goals for the immediate future. With the *Metabolize* program in mind, what are the specific improvements you want to make and all the reasons you want to succeed? Perhaps they've changed as you've been reading this book. But take a few minutes to define or redefine them. For example:

✔ "I want to lose twenty pounds. This will make me feel better about myself and give me more self-confidence."

✔ "I need to stop feeling so exhausted during the day. When I'm at work, I'm sometimes so run-down that I can't concentrate."

✔ "I'm starting to feel aches and pains throughout my body. I've got to get control of them before they begin to consume my life."

As part of the process of strengthening your attitude, take stock of your circumstances and set some priorities. Don't hesitate to dream a little. Of course, you shouldn't be naïve and create unrealistic expectations about this program and what it can accomplish; for example, don't count on an *overnight* transformation of your weight. But if you establish some goals and priorities, you'll have a much better chance of success—and a greater likelihood that those dreams will come true. That's what we'll try to accomplish in this chapter and the one that follows.

What are your priorities? Is one of them to make significant improvements in the way you feel? If so, you need to make a commitment to change the status quo. Think about what you're willing to do, each and every day, to turn that priority into a reality. Is altering your eating habits an important change you're willing to make? What about finding time to improve your breathing? Or performing the Seven No-Sweat Energy Movements?

As these priorities come together, they will help create the positive attitude you need. You'll feel yourself becoming more enthusiastic and excited about *Metabolize*. Remember, you are *not* doomed to live a life of being overweight, exhausted, and ill. Much more is within your control than you might imagine.

Of course, you may have to change some of your beliefs, which can be challenging. If you've always thought of yourself as a "fat" person, you still might see yourself that way even after you've lost weight. If you were a sickly child, you may feel that you're destined to remain that way for the rest of your life. But it's time to eliminate that "stinkin' thinkin.'" Look deeply within, and determine which beliefs you need to change. Then consciously adopt a *new* belief that's incompatible with the old one. If you've been sick and have believed that your chances of recovery are slim,

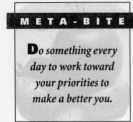

META-BITE

Do something every day to work toward your priorities to make a better you.

at least acknowledge the possibility that you can turn your health around. Better yet, recognize that the elements of this program have the power to make you *much* healthier. Become more open-minded about what you can accomplish. Create a new reality by choosing new beliefs. The odds of success really can turn in your favor.

IS SELF-TALK YOUR GREATEST SABOTEUR?

Sometimes we're our own worst enemies. All day long, we're talking to ourselves, and some of the messages aren't very appealing. Listen carefully to yourself. Do you sometimes hear things like:

- ✔ "Gee, I'm so fat."
- ✔ "Why can't I get off my rear end and exercise?"
- ✔ "I'm such a failure!"
- ✔ "It's my lousy genetics!"
- ✔ "I hate myself for the way I look!"

You can probably make a list of your own. Most of us maintain a constant inner dialogue. It plays and then replays as though it were on a continuous tape, and it's often not particularly friendly. Over many months and years, it can instill quite a negative self-image.

Where does this negative self-talk come from? Some of it may date back to childhood, when we were eliminated from a spelling bee or struck out in a softball game, or something was said to us by an unthinking adult ("You're never going to amount to anything!"). Although these experiences may have happened decades ago, they can have a lingering and devastating effect. There may be no present reality to support those impressions, but they can continue to shake our confidence and sabotage our best efforts in programs such as this one.

See if this rings true: As adults, many people tie their self-worth to the bathroom scale. Perhaps when you weigh more than you'd like, you feel absolutely worthless. You might compare yourself to the anorexic-slim women in fashion magazines and on billboards. ("Why aren't I as skinny as she? What's wrong with me?") And because our culture places such a stigma on overweight people, it's no wonder that negative self-talk becomes all-consuming whenever you gain a few pounds or see a little extra paunch when you look in the mirror.

Not surprisingly, your internal chatter can add plenty of stress to your life. If your boss unexpectedly throws a couple new assignments on your desk, you can react by saying, "I hate the way this office operates!!" and "Why does he always pick on me?" This response only compounds the stress. Or when you're stuck in a long supermarket checkout line, you might tell yourself, "This waiting is driving me absolutely crazy; it's going to make me late for my dinner tonight!"

You can reduce your stress levels, however, by changing your response to the situation. What if you just let the stress slide off your back? What if you changed your self-talk to say, "No big deal. I'll call my wife and tell her that the market is crowded and I'm running a little late."

ACCENTUATE THE NEGATIVE?

I sometimes ask clients to perform the following exercise, and I'd like you to do it as well. It's rather easy. Simply write down five *negative* beliefs you have about yourself that are part of your self-talk. Take a few moments to complete this exercise.

1. _____

2. _____

3. _____

4. _____

5. _____

What did you write? Were you able to come up with five? Some people have no difficulty thinking of negative things they say about themselves. They find it much harder to come up with *positive* statements.

What happens when you belittle yourself this way? It becomes part of your belief system. It sabotages your self-confidence. It creates anxiety and reduces your ability to succeed in programs like *Metabolize*.

That's why it's important to directly confront your negative self-talk and turn it into what I call Performance Talk. This is a technique that ensures that your self-talk becomes an ally, not an obstacle.

UNLEASHING PERFORMANCE TALK

To begin, think again about the negative inner dialogue that may run through your mind. This is the self-sabotaging thinking that may have made it difficult for you to succeed in weight-loss programs. It can provide insights into how you feel about yourself.

Really listen to yourself in this negative self-talk. Pay attention to just how critical, judgmental, and self-deprecating it is. If you say things like "I look disgusting!" or "No one could ever love someone this fat!" what kind of message are you sending to your subconscious mind?

Too often, this internal chatter nags at us. It becomes a constant reminder of our limitations and shortcomings, real or imagined. It is brutal, unfriendly, and certainly not in your best interest. Most distressing, this self-talk can become a self-fulfilling prophecy. For example, if you're inundated with thoughts such as "I'll never succeed with this program," you probably won't! And you just might reach for a couple brownies to make yourself feel better!

For *Metabolize* to work, you need to change your self-talk. You can't control what other people are saying or thinking, but you have *complete* control over your own mind and inner dialogue.

With your self-talk in mind, ask yourself, "Is what I'm saying true?" It sometimes helps to repeat those negative statements slowly. Say them aloud and exaggerate each word. Are they really based in reality? What irrefutable evidence do you have that these things are true?

You might not be consciously aware of the powerful influence that negative self-talk is having upon your life. You might slip into a rut and get stuck in it as though it were quicksand. I lived in Nebraska for nine years, and sometimes I could drive on a country road with my tires in a rut or groove in the road that was caused by the wheels of thousands of cars passing over it so many times that the road actually sank a little. I could literally remove my hands from the steering wheel and the car would continue straight down the road without even the slightest bit of weaving; it was as though I were on a ride at Disneyland, traveling on an inescapable track. The only way to escape from the rut on those Nebraska roads was to make a concerted effort to take back control of the steering wheel, turning it to the left or the right and freeing my car from the groove.

That's exactly what you need to do with your negative self-talk. You have complete control over your thinking. So grasp the steering wheel and turn self-talk into a positive force in your life. *Metabolize* is taking you down a new road. Leave your old baggage behind so it doesn't weigh you down.

Performance Talk uses positive statements to elevate you above your negative thoughts and surround you with an environment of excellence that supports your health and lifestyle goals. It is quality thinking that conditions the mind and reinforces your personal strengths and ties them to positive emotions.

Here's one way to think about Performance Talk. Imagine turning on a faucet, with its stream of clean water directed into a glass filled with dirty water. As the faucet water pours into the glass, it gradually displaces the dirty water. Before long, there is no dirty water left in the glass. In the same way, Performance Talk saturates your mind with positive messages, leaving no room for negative ones. When that happens, you can dramatically transform your beliefs about yourself.

Performance Talk puts a positive slant on the thoughts that are already spinning through your mind. For example:

> Negative self-talk: "Geez, I have so much more weight to lose; I'm still such a slob!"
>
> Performance Talk: "I am already eight pounds lighter, and I am on track to lose all the weight I want to."

The concept is pretty simple. You're removing the negative and replacing it with the positive. Sure, you're still aware of your weaknesses; we all have them. But you're accentuating the positive, which really can become a supportive influence over time.

One strategy is to take your negative self-talk and reframe it so that it has a positive slant. It takes your imperfections and positions them in a way that encourages your strengths to flourish. Let me give you an example. I'm not a particularly organized person. But in my self-talk, I could approach this "shortcoming" in two ways:

NEGATIVE SELF-TALK: "I'm so disorganized! Why can't I do anything right?"

PERFORMANCE TALK: "I am not the most organized person in the world, but a little disorganization actually allows me to be creative."

Not long ago, I worked with a world-class pole vaulter named Dean Starkey. As a vaulter, he participates in the most dangerous and demanding track and field event; it requires speed, strength, and enormous courage. Without a doubt, Dean is one of the best, finishing second in the World Championships in 1997. But when we began working together, he had vaulted over the 19-foot barrier only once. No attempt after that ever exceeded the 19-foot height. He felt frustrated and exasperated. "It must have been a fluke," he told himself. "I must have gotten lucky once."

I knew it was important to transform Dean's self-talk. I told him, "You were able to vault nineteen feet once. You can do it again. You're just twenty-five years old. You're in your prime. You should be reaching your peak now. Your self-talk needs to change from 'It was a fluke' to 'I am capable of vaulting nineteen feet again and again.'"

Dean made a conscious effort to alter his inner dialogue. He started reconditioning his mind: "I am capable of vaulting nineteen feet . . . I am capable of vaulting nineteen feet. . . ." He used that Performance Talk, day after day, week after week.

In the subsequent year, how did Dean vault? He cleared the bar at 19 feet *five times.* Not bad! In the process, his world ranking soared as well, climbing from number seven to number two. Pretty impressive for someone who once believed that his best vault was a "fluke."

Performance Talk is a phrase or statement, and a way of affirming that you can soar to the next level. It is as powerful as a prescription medication ordered by your doctor. When I work with people who are trying to improve their health and/or lose pounds, I have them focus their Performance Talk so it speaks to the way they'd like to be in the weeks and months ahead. They might say things like:

✔ "I am healthy and weigh 125 pounds."
✔ "I am healthy and love exercise."

✔ "I am calm and centered because I belly breathe."
✔ "I am making informed, intelligent decisions about the food I eat."
✔ "I am healthy, happy, and fulfilled."

Notice that these statements are positive and support your success in the *Metabolize* program. By using Performance Talk to frame your life as you'd like it to become, you're giving your mind a road to travel along.

Bear in mind, however, that negative thoughts are okay only *if* they lead to positive action. I sometimes tell the story of Positive Paul and Marvelous Mary, standing in their underwear in their front yard in the midst of a Minnesota blizzard. With goofy grins on their faces, they proclaim, "We *love* the cold," as if they're on a sunny beach in Florida. Sure, they're thinking positively, but before long their grins will become frozen in place. For them, it would be better to have a negative thought ("I hate the cold! I'm miserable!") that leads to positive action ("We're freezing! Let's go in the house, call our travel agent, and head for Florida!").

Performance Talk is designed to lead to positive action. So pause a moment, and write down five Performance Talk statements. These are positive pronouncements that you believe to be true about yourself—or that you believe *can* become true with the guidance of *Metabolize*. They are issues that you want to focus on and improve. This kind of positive self-talk often works best when the words are in the present tense, particularly statements that begin with, "I am . . .".

1. _____

2. _____

3. _____

4. _____

5. _____

Once you create your Performance Talk statement(s), write them on a three-by-five card. Refer back to them several times a day. (Some people look at them every morning and night.) Repeat them to yourself during the day with passion and belief. As you say them, see them. As you see them, feel them.

Repeat your Performance Talk statements when you're in the supermarket, making choices about the most appropriate food to bring home.

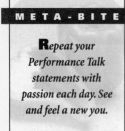

META-BITE

Repeat your Performance Talk statements with passion each day. See and feel a new you.

Say them when you're home, opening the refrigerator and making decisions that will influence your health.

Performance Talk is one of the easiest and fastest ways to change your belief system. You have more strength and power than you realize. Use it to support yourself in this program.

Remember, everything starts in the mind first. Self-talk can enhance your health or undermine it. It can support high performance, or it can become a self-destructive force that sends you into a downward spiral. You have the ability to break the negative life cycles in which you might find yourself. The choice is yours.

THOSE INEVITABLE LAPSES . . .

So you've made a commitment to this program and are already beginning to change your eating and other health-related habits, or you are at least making plans for those changes. Or perhaps by now you're enjoying some early progress with *Metabolize.* But what happens if something throws you out of sync? Perhaps you'll see an entrée on a restaurant menu that's one of your favorites but not a good choice for your Metabolic Type—and you give in to the temptation. You order the item and enjoy it thoroughly but feel absolutely terrible afterward. Virtually overnight, you believe that all is lost. You revert back to your old behaviors. Before long, it is as though you had never been on the program at all.

Keep this important point in mind: No matter how conscientiously you try to adhere to the *Metabolize* program, there *will* be times when you slip. Perhaps during a period of enormous stress at work, or when you're coping with a serious family illness, you won't eat the way you should. Or you may wait too long between meals and in response to your hunger, you may make poor food choices. Or maybe you'll skip your daily workout sessions, or find your breathing out of sorts.

Your ability to cope with lapses depends largely on what we've been discussing throughout this chapter—your attitude. If you acknowledge now that from time to time, you'll experience these lapses, you'll have the positive frame of mind to immediately rebound.

Too often, people become overwhelmed by these slips. They throw up their hands, announce to themselves, "You've failed again!" and go back to their old (and problematic) ways of managing their health. But you need to be kinder to yourself. Yes, you may have made what seemed like a poor choice, but at the time, it was actually the "best" choice, perhaps meeting an emotional need that you had at that moment. By being prepared for these inevitable lapses and knowing that life is filled with both peaks and valleys, you won't get down on yourself, and you'll be better able to effectively rebound from these disruptions and keep them to a minimum in the future.

Nobody's perfect. So make a conscious decision to forgive yourself and work through reversals when they occur. Shift your attitude so you stay one step ahead of the lapses, and when they happen, grow from them. Refocus on the important components of this program, and get back on track. That kind of "take control" outlook will serve you well.

After a slip, make an effort to become more conscious of the food choices you make. Before each meal, ask yourself questions like:

✔ What food(s) will satisfy me right now?
✔ Will this choice contribute to reaching my ideal weight?
✔ Is there a better choice I can make today to ensure good health in the future?

Also, keep your sense of humor. Learn to laugh at yourself and your shortcomings. When people ask how they can tell when they're overweight, I sometimes quip, "Forget about the bathroom scale! Stand naked in front of a full-length mirror, and then jump in the air as high as you can. When you land, look at your body in the mirror. If it's still moving after thirty seconds, you need to lose some weight!"

With your sense of humor intact, you won't become devastated by those inevitable lapses. And you'll find that if you return to *Metabolize* as soon as possible, those slips will become less frequent over time. That's because this program will make you feel like a new person. The temptations that lead to lapses will become much less appealing because you won't want to give back any of the progress you've made. You'll love what you see when you look at yourself in the mirror. You'll experience the difference. You'll want to hold on to to it. As you'll discover, health does feel much better than illness.

Meta-Check

What if you find yourself wanting to go back to unhealthy habits? How can you stay on track? Here are some strategies to try:

➜ Check to make sure you are eating primarily from your Preferred list.

➜ Monitor your ratios—they matter!

➜ Try a meditation or belly-breathing exercise, and ask yourself, "What do I really want?"

➜ Make sure you're doing the Seven No-Sweat Energy Movements regularly.

➜ If you splurge, take notice of how you feel afterward. Remember, there is no failure—only feedback.

➜ Confide in a friend who has a positive outlook. For some people, prayer helps.

➜ Consider getting your own *Metabolize* coach with whom you can communicate via phone, e-mail, or letter. Contact the Biodynamics Institute at 1-800-828-3343 or on the Internet at *www.metabolize.net.*

11

Balanced Body, Balanced Mind

No matter what your hopes for this program were when you started reading—perhaps to lose weight or maybe to improve your overall health—you now have the tools to reach those goals. This is a commonsense, practical program in which I've asked you to concentrate on a number of important areas—eating, breathing, moving, and thinking. When you do so, and do it conscientiously, I'm confident that you'll lead a longer, healthier life.

In this chapter, I'll add the final component of this program—namely, the importance of bringing balance to your body and mind. I'll help you elevate your values into your conscious awareness and, as that happens, make them the guiding forces in your life.

YOUR HIERARCHY OF VALUES

Good health, as I define it, is much more than the absence of disease. It also involves living in accordance with your core values—those deep-seated beliefs that mean everything to you.

Something unfortunate happens to most people; maybe you've noticed it happening to you. The dreams and the values that they once thought would always guide them somehow slipped into a subordinate role. They became so caught up in the pressing demands of day-to-day life that their values were forgotten and their dreams were postponed. It happens to so many people. But it shouldn't be that way.

To have good health, your life needs to be in balance. To be truly healthy, you need to elevate your values to a place of prominence in your life and let them guide you. Losing 25 pounds is fine, but it won't make you feel that much better if your personal relationships are in chaos, and you're not the spouse or the parent that you once dreamed of being. Incorporating the Seven No-Sweat Energy Movements into your daily routine is important, but it won't have nearly the impact that it could if your spiritual needs were being met. Having more energy may help you get through the day, but it won't soothe the anguish you feel sitting at your desk at work, knowing that you're spending your life at a job that you no longer enjoy, looking forward to little more than those moments when you say, "Thank God it's Friday!"

I've known people who genuinely believe that their life is getting better, year by year. (I'm very fortunate to be one of them.) These individuals get excited just thinking about the future. They are driven by their dreams. They are faithful to their values. They have clearly defined goals that strongly influence most of the decisions in their lives.

Do these descriptions fit you? Or do you fall into the following category instead: Over time, have most or all of your aspirations turned into "impossible dreams"? Have you lost the hope of achieving true self-fulfillment? Whether you are a high school dropout or have a Ph.D., make deals on Wall Street or flip burgers at McDonald's, been married for 20 years or divorced six months after you tied the knot, perhaps your life just isn't right. And you know it.

WHAT ARE YOUR CORE VALUES?

Even though it's easy to lose sight of your values, you need to reposition them as a primary motivational force in your life. They should be the principles that you want your life to stand for.

YOUR HIERARCHY OF VALUES

I've conducted this exercise with hundreds of clients one on one and with thousands of people at seminars. It has helped them elevate their values into their consciousness and truly reconnect with them. It is a first step toward making some important life choices about their future.

Using the chart below, write down the ten most important values in your life. Don't think for hours about what they are. Just turn your attention to the task at hand; allow them to come to mind without effort. Don't judge whether they really belong on your list. Simply follow your heart, and write down what comes forth. Although you might find yourself stuck after coming up with four or five, keep going; extend the list to ten if you can. Don't worry about the order in which you list them. Just commit them to paper, one after the other.

1. _____
2. _____
3. _____
4. _____
5. _____
6. _____
7. _____
8. _____
9. _____
10. _____

Once you've completed your list, review it carefully. Then, in the second part of this exercise, I'd like you to rearrange your list, this time placing the values in their order of importance, from 1 to 10. In essence ask yourself, "Which of these values do I hold in the highest esteem?" Go ahead and do this in the space that follows:

1. _____
2. _____
3. _____

4. _____

5. _____

6. _____

7. _____

8. _____

9. _____

10. _____

What values rose to the top of your list? A devotion to God and your faith? A commitment to your family and friends? The importance of a strong and intimate marriage? The value of good health? A commitment to building your career? The importance of personal integrity? Of compassion? Of education and learning? The value of service to others? The need for having a financially secure future?

Look at your Hierarchy of Values frequently. As you do, ask yourself questions like these:

- ✔ "Am I really getting what I want out of life?
- ✔ "Am I really *living* my primary values?"
- ✔ "How do I spend each day—not only doing the things I *have* to do, but how do I spend my free time?"
- ✔ "What should I be spending more of my time doing?"
- ✔ "What kind of person am I right now, and who would I like to become in the future?"
- ✔ "What would bring more fulfillment and balance into my life?"

At age 32, Benjamin Franklin examined his own life and his values, then made some decisions on where he would devote his energies in the future. He wrote, "Be a better father . . . be a better husband . . . be financially independent . . . improve my mind . . . be temperate."

Many other admirable historical figures—from Mohandas Gandhi to Martin Luther King, Jr.—consciously defined their own values and then remained true to them. It changed their lives, and the lives of many other people.

GET SMART!

Now your Hierarchy of Values is in place. Next, you should set goals and create a state of mind to support them. You need to do more than just hope that your life will fall into place the way you want it to. You should know exactly where you'd like to go before you start. You must take action to ensure that your values become part of your everyday life.

As part of the goal-setting process, keep the acronym *SMART* in mind:

✔ **Specific.** You need to be specific and clear about how you want your life to evolve. Know what you want to accomplish in the weeks, months, and years ahead. What do you want your health to be like? What about your family life? Your career? Your financial status? You can begin to mold your future by establishing goals that reflect your values clearly, without any ambiguity. Instead of saying, "I'd like to get my health to improve," change it to "I will get my cholesterol to a level below 200 so I can stop taking that cholesterol-lowering drug."

✔ **Measurable.** When you measure a goal, you give it a sense of urgency and it can help you keep track of how you're progressing. Do you want to reshape your diet so that your carbohydrate-protein-fat ratio is 60%/20%/20%? Or should it be 40%/30%/30%? Set the goal with precision. For example, I worked with a college basketball player whose dream was to play his sport to the best of his potential. At the time, he was shooting free throws at a 70 percent rate but he wanted to improve to 85 percent. So he set measurable interim goals—to improve to 72 percent after two weeks, 75 percent after four weeks, and so on. He kept his enthusiasm level high by reaching each one of these minigoals, and eventually he was shooting slightly *better* than 85 percent!

✔ **Attainable.** Make your target a reachable one. While weight loss may be your primary goal with the *Metabolize* program, it may *not* be realistic to lose 25 pounds during the first 21 days of this program. *No* plan can legitimately promise that kind of rapid weight loss. So make sure you're setting goals that are achievable, and that you're willing to make the sacrifices necessary to reach them. (For example, are you inclined to do what it takes to stick with this program for 42 days?)

✔ **Realistic.** None of us can transform ourselves into Superman or Wonder Woman. Nor can most of us ever look like Twiggy. (Nor should we want to!) Sure, it's good to shoot for the stars and set lofty goals. But while these goals can be challenging, you'll only be setting yourself up for disappointment if they're unrealistic. To determine if your goal is realistic, ask yourself, "Has anyone achieved this before?" If someone has (or if you truly believe you can be the first)—and you're willing to work hard and pay the price to get there—go for it!

✔ **Time-driven.** Set a definite deadline to reach a particular goal. The first phase of this program is 21 days long, and thus a time frame is built right into it. When you know that you have a time frame in which to make something happen, you will often find yourself much better focused and more strongly committed.

MY GOALS

Now take a few minutes to set some goals for yourself. Make sure they are supportive of and in sync with your own Hierarchy of Values. Don't worry about the order in which you write them down. Just commit these goals to paper below:

1. _____
2. _____
3. _____
4. _____
5. _____
6. _____
7. _____
8. _____
9. _____
10. _____

As you're setting goals, also be sure to answer the question, "Why do I want to achieve them?" If they reflect your values, that's all the reason you need.

Next, select the top three goals from the list above. Rank them according to their importance. These are the primary goals you should focus on in the weeks ahead.

1. _____

2. _____

3. _____

What can you do to ensure that these goals become reality? Create some minigoals that inspire you—that is, baby steps or small shifts in behavior that can eventually produce large changes. This might mean using your leisure time more productively and paying more attention to what you watch, listen to, and read. It may require turning off the television at night and devoting more time to reading an enriching book or participating in family activities. It could mean putting aside the Sunday morning newspaper and going to church instead. It might require giving up your bowling league and spending that time taking night classes at a community college or meditating on your past successes. It may suggest listening to music that inspires you, or motivational tapes that boost your spirits. Each of these steps can be supportive of your overall well-being. Once you begin to live your life in harmony with your Hierarchy of Values, you'll finally experience your true potential.

During the course of this program and beyond, never lose sight of this Hierarchy of Values and the goals that can help you reach them. When appropriate, rework and rewrite them. Make sure they are still your values and your goals. And ask yourself whether you've made progress toward fulfilling them. Rather than giving them lip service, give them *life* service!

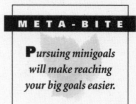

META-BITE

Pursuing minigoals will make reaching your big goals easier.

PEERING INTO THE FUTURE

To prepare the way for the 21-day program that will pull together all the components of *Metabolize*, let's try a technique called Future Pace that can preview what your life will be like when you are true to your Hierarchy of Values. This is a total sensory technique in which you will call upon all of your senses to experience today what your future will be like.

As you know, the brain has two hemispheres. They look the same to the human eye, but they function in very different ways. While the left hemisphere uses logic, analysis, rationality, and language, the right hemisphere processes its information through imagination and pictures. When you use visualization, your brain is active in the right hemisphere. These images can be extremely powerful and support the notion that "a picture is worth a thousand words."

Initially, I introduced Future Pace to athletes I was working with. After using it, they described it as the most powerful mental training exercise they had ever tried. As part of *Metabolize*, it will allow you to use the language of the right brain in a way where you'll be able to see, feel, and experience what it will be like to achieve your goals and live according to your Hierarchy of Values.

Some people find it helpful to slowly read the following exercise into a tape recorder, then play it back with their eyes shut. When you're ready, let's begin:

Sit in a comfortable chair. Close your eyes, take a deep breath, and exhale gently. Continue to breathe this way for another 30 seconds or so. . . .

Now, I'd like you to project yourself into the future, about six weeks from now, when you have completed this program. You have spent weeks conscientiously eating according to your Metabolic Type, performing the Seven No-Sweat Energy Movements, practicing proper breathing techniques, and developing a success-oriented attitude. . . .

Next, notice what it's like to have already achieved the goal(s) that brought you to this program in the first place. Perhaps you wanted to lose 15 pounds. So take a few moments now to look into a mirror, and see yourself with a better body and fitting comfortably into the clothes of your choice. Make your images as vivid as possible. . . . Notice the color of your clothes, the posture of your body, and the expression on your face.

Picture yourself in public settings, at work or at social occasions, and receiving compliments about the way you look. Experience the words of encouragement, the pats on the back, the high fives. . . . Notice the increased sense of self-confidence you feel, thanks to your commitment to the Metabolize *program. . . .*

Also, picture how you'll feel physically at the end of the program. . . . Notice how much more energy you have. . . . Become aware of the absence of any aches and pains that used to plague you. . . . Notice that your breathing is calmer and more relaxed than it has ever been. . . . Feel yourself being more in tune with your body thanks to the Seven No-Sweat Energy Movements. . . .

Become aware that you are much more active than you've been in a long time. . . . What is your body posture like? Feel yourself standing taller than usual, with your shoulders back. . . . Notice the happy and content expression on your face. Perhaps it's an irresistible, ear-to-ear smile. Or a picture of calmness and relaxation. . . . You certainly like what you see, don't you? . . . Experience the "new you" now. . . .

Think back on everything you did right to make these dramatic changes and improvements. . . . Become aware of how your values have a much stronger place in your life than they once did. . . . Look back at your successes on this program thus far, and tell yourself, "I did it!" Notice how it feels to say these words, the tone of your voice, and the success that you are experiencing.

As you enjoy the rewards of these accomplishments, ask yourself, "Was it worth it? Was it worth the dedication and the commitment that got me here?" And as you conclude that it was, start to work backward in time. . . . Notice some of the obstacles you had to overcome along the way to achieve your goals. . . . Observe the negative people whom you dealt with effectively. Remember what you said to counter their negativity. . . . Recall how you exercised even when you were tired, how you moved away from food temptations, and how you called upon inner strength to make positive changes in your life. . . .

Continue to work back in time, and examine where you had been when you started this quest. Notice how far you've come in just a few weeks. Allow yourself to experience satisfaction over what you've achieved. You've accomplished a lot . . . little things, big things. . . .

Just before opening your eyes, feel good about allowing your whole mind, your entire body, and all of your emotions to work together in harmony to make this happen. Realize that you have a compelling and exciting future. This is just the beginning.

Now you have a sense of what your success with this program will be like. You can see how your old destructive feelings of helplessness can be overcome, and what the amazing benefits will be. You have given your mind a path to follow. You are in control.

12

Getting Better Faster: Metabolizing Tips for Athletes

Not long ago, I began working with a 21-year-old athlete named David, who was competing on a Division I college swim team. He had been feeling discouraged for some time, believing that his peak swimming days were behind him. He was feeling pressure to win, but he doubted that he would ever get any better. His dejection affected many aspects of his life, not just watering down his performance in the pool but also propelling his academics into a dive. He frequently complained of feeling worn down and burned out. "Swimming," he said, "just isn't fun anymore."

At one point, David seriously considered quitting the swim team. But then he had a change of heart. "I don't want to set a precedent in my life of quitting when things get tough," he said. David's coach referred him to me, hoping that I might be able to get him back on track.

Initially, David and I concentrated on the mental side of his sport. I had worked with hundreds of athletes by that time, including many swimmers, and felt confident that by stretching his mind, I could help David; after just a few sessions, I believed, he'd be back in the pool, more successful than ever. But, boy, was I wrong! David's attitude did improve dramatically, but his performance in the pool remained waterlogged. It was a real mystery. After all, his training program was very solid, designed by two of the best swimming coaches in the area. I helped him create some time-management strategies, which helped extricate him from those out-of-control feelings of drowning in his schoolwork, training sessions, and social life—but he still wasn't swimming any faster. Even though David was at an age where male athletes are still maturing physically, he seemed to have dropped anchor and wasn't making any forward progress. It was a frustrating situation.

What was left? Finally, we began analyzing David's diet. He ate like many other middle-distance swimmers—plenty of carbohydrates and limited fats and proteins. It was a healthy diet, but it wasn't working for David. So working together, we determined his Metabolic Type (Clean), and then I suggested changes in his diet: More protein, a little more fat, fewer carbohydrates.

I checked back with David about two weeks later. Wow! Things were dramatically different, he said, and it was all positive. His energy levels had soared. He was thinking much more clearly. He found it easier to concentrate on his schoolwork. And what about his performance in the pool? "My endurance is much, much better," he told me. "And I've started swimming faster, actually beating the times I had been stuck on for so long!" There was genuine joy in David's voice. And, yes, he said that the changes in his diet seemed to make all the difference.

During his junior year, David won many races. He continued to exceed his fastest times. "Swimming," he said, "is finally fun again."

Athletes have played a major role in the development of *Metabolize*. In many years as a sports performance consultant, I fine-tuned this program not only with college-level swimmers like David but also with professional football, basketball, and baseball players, pro soccer and beach volleyball players, and hundreds of high school athletes. In nearly 90 percent of them, *Metabolize* produced fast, positive results in their performance. If you play sports, whether on a community softball team or on the U.S. Olympic team, you can do the same.

WHAT ABOUT PROTEIN?

All athletes serious about improving their game should become sensitive to their metabolic individuality. They need to identify their Metabolic Type and then adopt the optimal diet for it. But that may not be all. They may also need to make additional nutritional adjustments. Most commonly, their protein requirements might increase, which also necessitates a change in the amount of carbohydrates and fats that they consume.

Let's say that you participate in a sport where you're trying to build muscle mass. If you're a Clean or Super-Clean metabolizer, the ratios for your type (described in Chapter 5) should be just fine. Your diet already calls for large amounts of protein and more modest levels of carbohydrates and fat. If you do decide to experiment with raising your protein consumption, do so very modestly.

On the other hand, if you're a Super-Lean, Lean, or Mixed metabolizer, you are eating on the lower end of the protein spectrum. As an athlete, you may have greater protein needs than a sedentary person, so your body can build and repair muscle tissue; thus you may need to increase your protein consumption, which will help boost your muscle mass.

Here's my suggestion: If your Type is Super-Lean, and you're an athlete, you'll achieve better performance by shifting your nutrient ratio to that of the Lean metabolizer—that is, rather than eating a 70% carbohydrate/15% protein/15% fat diet, change to one with 60% carbohydrate/20% protein/20% fat. Even though athletes really get very little energy from protein (most comes from carbohydrates and fat), your body will benefit from the extra protein (and fat) in your diet; 15 percent is simply not enough for someone who is very physically active.

Now, if you're a Lean or Mixed metabolizer, my advice is a little different: *Don't* alter your ratio—stick with the one for your Type—but add more protein to your diet by increasing your overall caloric content a little and at the same time raising your carbohydrate and fat intake as well. Thus, you'll be eating more protein—and more carbohydrate and fat—but keeping them in the same ratio as described in Chapter 5.

Frankly, all athletes, no matter what their Type, need to be aware of the protein content of their diet. An endurance runner—or even a construction worker doing strenuous work all day—has a voracious need for protein that needs to be replenished. If that doesn't happen, the body will begin to "cannibalize" its own muscle to obtain more protein. The result: Muscle breakdown and fatigue, and a greater chance of injury.

Some athletes meet their need for extra protein by eating a protein-rich food bar. If you decide to go that route, choose one manufactured by a reputable company; read its label carefully, looking for a nutrient ratio that closely matches the ratio for your Metabolic Type. A Lean metabolizer should be thinking about adding about one ounce of protein to his or her diet with each snack. Use the same approach when selecting a protein supplement (a protein drink or powder); for maximum benefits, it should contain nutrients as near to your own optimal ratio as possible.

But keep the following in mind: As I pointed out in Chapter 6, the body can utilize only about 40 grams or so of protein per meal. Thus, while you may need to increase your overall protein intake to provide your body with everything it requires, don't overdo it. You need to find and maintain a balance of nutrients. Too much protein over long periods of time can overwork your kidneys and excretory system to the point of causing serious organ damage. Excess protein can also cause a loss of calcium in your bones (via the urine) and increase the risk of dehydration (as your body utilizes water to excrete protein).

How can you tell if you're consuming too much protein? The simplest indicator is that you'll begin urinating more often when you change your diet. Or your urine may develop a strong ammonialike smell.

One other important point: Unlike other programs that place nearly all of their emphasis on protein, *Metabolize* takes a much more well-rounded approach. Its balanced nutritional system provides fuel for all three key energy systems of the body that athletes rely on (called the *immediate, glycolytic,* and *oxidative* energy systems). Thus, whether your particular sport requires energy for explosive, short-term movements or for endurance activities, a foundation of *Metabolize* should meet your needs.

SPECIAL SUPPLEMENTS: DO THEY MAKE SENSE?

If you're an athlete, multivitamin-multimineral pills may be even more important than for the nonathlete, because of the unusual physical stress to which you're routinely subjecting your body.

But should you be taking anything else? What about all of the other supplements aimed at athletes? Walk through any health food store, and you'll see shelves packed with a mind-boggling array of pills and potions. Some promise to build muscle mass. Others insist that they can increase endurance. They all make amazing performance-enhancing claims. Frankly, if you added up all the promises, you'd see the glint of an Olympic gold medal in your future.

With many of these pills, there's much more hype than proven benefits. Here are my recommendations about some of the currently popular pills:

✔ Protein supplements are an effective way to increase your protein intake (although food, not pills, is the optimal source of protein). But if you're trying to increase your protein intake, particularly between meals, consider giving these protein supplements a try. They are effective for many people and are cost-efficient.

✔ Creatine became the hottest supplement for athletes in the late 1990s and has been promoted primarily as a builder of rippling muscles. In fact, many power lifters, football linemen, and other strength athletes have joined the creatine craze and have reported positive results.

Creatine is an amino acid stored in muscle tissue. It replenishes the compound called adenosine triphosphate (ATP), which is the source of energy used by muscles during physical activity. Creatine may be able to fire up muscles for explosive bursts of energy and accelerate recovery from vigorous exercise. But consider this important caveat: There are *no* long-term studies of creatine's benefits and, perhaps more importantly, of its possible risks to organs like the heart, liver, and kidneys. I have read anecdotal reports that creatine has caused muscle pulls and tears and has contributed to dehydration. Some users have complained of minor side effects such as nausea, diarrhea, and cramps. So give some thought to the possible downside before you begin popping creatine pills with regularity.

✔ Steroidlike supplements, particularly androstenedione, received an enormous amount of publicity when home-run king Mark McGwire acknowledged using them in his memorable drive toward 70 home runs in 1998. These products are sold over the counter, but they have some of the same physiological effects as anabolic steroids.

Androstenedione is a hormone produced naturally in the body in small amounts, and it stimulates muscle growth. But when consumed as a supplement, it alters the body's natural hormonal balance; the liver converts androstenedione into testosterone, which helped produce McGwire's Popeye-sized biceps. But the use of these supplements worries me; it must also concern the National Football League, the National Collegiate Athletic Association, and the International Olympic Committee, all of which have banned them. The Association of Professional Team Physicians has recommended that they be removed from the marketplace.

Androstenedione was developed in East Germany, where athletes (mostly women) took it. Yes, it appears to be safe short-term for most people, but no one knows what its long-term side effects may be. It just hasn't been studied well enough. There is some worry that too much testosterone can cause everything from acne and increased aggressiveness to baldness and breast development in men, as well as the stunting of bone growth and heart and liver problems. It now appears that androstenedione increases levels of the female hormone estrogen, which in men can lead to enlarged breasts, an increased risk of certain cancers (of the pancreas, for example), and a decline in HDL ("good") cholesterol, placing them at a greater risk of heart attacks or stroke. That's what happens when you play around with hormones. And for every Mark McGwire whose body seems to handle androstenedione well, there may be another person for whom there could be serious negative effects. I suggest staying away from it, particularly if you're a teenager still growing. If you do decide to try it, never exceed the manufacturer's dosage recommendations.

Remember, as an athlete, your nutritional (particularly protein) needs could differ a little from those of a sedentary person. But if you increase your protein intake, keep your overall dietary ratio in sync with your Metabolic Type. Eating in accordance with your Type should give you a big head start in the competitive arena. Athletes can contact the Biodynamics Institute for a customized nutrition and supplement program.

13

The 21-Day Action Plan

> "Knowledge is a treasure chest,
> action is the key."
>
> —ANONYMOUS

There is a story about a treasure hunter who spent weeks upgrading the condition of his boat and outfitting it with new equipment. He hired a five-man crew, and they set off from shore. Their mission: to find buried treasure.

Sure enough, within two days, they had located an aging chest on the ocean floor, presumed to be filled with jewels. They rejoiced, and the liquor flowed freely. As they continued to congratulate each other on their discovery, they pulled the chest onto the deck of the boat. As they formed a circle around it, what do you think they did next? Did they simply stare at the unopened chest and then lower it back into the sea?

Get real! The treasure hunter didn't spend all those weeks preparing for the journey at sea just to go through the motions of finding and then discarding the chest without ever opening it. Realizing the potential riches that awaited him, he broke open the lock and lifted the lid. And in fact, he did find jewels inside—lots of jewels. There were enough to finance an entire fleet of boats for his next treasure-hunting expedition. He had struck it rich!

In the same way, this book is filled with riches of a different kind. In it, you've found a treasure chest of information that can literally transform your life for the better. It can turn your health around and put you on course to shed all the weight you want to lose. So let me congratulate you on reading this far and absorbing a lot of important information.

But of course, you need to do more than just read this book. Simply acquainting yourself with this program isn't enough; that alone won't translate into improvements in your well-being. I'm sure you know that.

So if you haven't already done so, now it's time to take the plunge. You need to decide whether you're only going to stare at the treasure chest in this book, or whether you're going to do much more—extract its value and actively use what you've learned.

I have seen the *Metabolize* program dramatically change the lives of so many of my own clients. Now you can join them. Remember, weight loss—as well as optimal health and longevity—are dependent on an efficiently functioning metabolism that maximizes energy production at the cellular level. But for that to happen, you need to make and keep a commitment to take full advantage of what you've found in these pages. Yes, it takes some effort to achieve peak metabolism—although that effort can reap benefits tenfold by normalizing your body weight and improving your overall well-being.

This chapter will provide you with a 21-Day Action Plan times 2. In other words, you need to stick with this plan for 42 days—and here's why. The brain is very powerful, and the right mindset is vital to the success of this program. As I pointed out in Chapter 10, however, research shows that motivation lasts only 17 days (give or take a few days either way). So while your initial excitement for *Metabolize* will carry you through most or all of the first three weeks, it really takes six weeks, or 42 days, for this program to fully alter your internal chemistry for long-term change. So a 42-day or six-week plan is your actual target.

Can you stick with it for 42 days? Almost everyone I've worked with has. The good news is that this program does not require any superhuman sacrifices. You won't find it to be terribly restrictive. It's not all-consuming. Focus completely on the first 21 days right now. Most people on *Metabolize* begin to feel the first positive results within the first few days. When that happens, it helps keep them enthusiastic for the long term. It will stimulate excitement that can motivate them right through the second 21 days.

So start creating a vision now of 21 days. You can do it. And when you do, you will begin to experience all of the benefits of this program.

Keep in mind that you have your own biochemical individuality that needs to be addressed. With a nutritional plan cus-tomized for your unique metabolism, plus the other key components of this program, you *can* reach your weight-loss and other health goals. Better yet, those changes can become permanent. You won't have to suffer. You won't feel deprived. And the Action Plan in this chapter will give you the structure to turn your goals into reality.

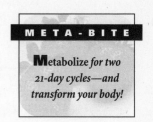

META-BITE

Metabolize *for two 21-day cycles—and transform your body!*

MAKING THE COMMITMENT

This program can work wonders, but only if you promise to stick with it for two consecutive 21-day cycles. You'll need to focus on the first three weeks, then refocus on the next three.

Are you ready to make a strong commitment to this 21-days-times-2 program? Are you willing to put it in writing? This is a very important first step in your Action Plan. By signing the "contract" below, you can ac-tually strengthen your resolve. A written agreement carries much more power than a verbal one.

My own clients have told me that when moments of self-doubt sur-faced, they found it much more difficult to turn tail and run for cover when this contract was in front of them. As one young woman said, "Of course, it doesn't carry any legal weight, but you'd be surprised at the inner strength it gave me."

So write your name and sign your contract. At the same time, choose a date to start this program. Don't wait for the "perfect time" to get started. Take action now! Once you've decided on a starting date, add it to your agreement. The important thing is to commit yourself to get started and to see it through. So set a date. Then get ready for 42 days that can dramatically improve your life!

I, _____ , pledge to use *Metabolize*
        (your name)

for two consecutive 21-day cycles. I will begin the program on the date below.

        Signed,

        _____

        Starting date: _____

WHAT ARE YOUR HEALTH GOALS?

To keep your motivation as strong as possible during the 21-Day Action Plan times 2, you can't lose sight of the person you want to become by Day 42. In Chapter 11, when we discussed bringing balance into your life, I asked you to think about and write down your own Hierarchy of Values. They might have included a strong marriage, a good education, nurturing your family life, building a rewarding career, and developing compassion and personal integrity. Hopefully, good health was one of your values as well. In fact, if good health was on your list—and is a value you live by—it can serve as a foundation that keeps you energetic and makes reaching *all* of your goals possible.

Sit back and take a few moments now to think about the importance of good health and how you'd like to improve yours. In your own mind, contemplate what you really want in terms of your well-being, now and in the future. Dream big, but with this caveat: Keep your dreams within the realm of reality. If you hope to turn yourself into the next *Sports Illustrated* swimsuit model, that may not be a realistic dream (although perhaps it could be). If you picture yourself modeling Calvin Klein underwear or winning a part on *Baywatch*, consider the possibility that fame and fortune aren't necessarily at the end of your *Metabolize* rainbow (but maybe they are). If you want to run a ten-kilometer race in 36 minutes, that may simply be too fast for your own body. While it's fine to set your sights high, you're much more likely to reach goals that are real, genuine, and relevant to your life and body type.

When I asked a woman named Linda about her aspirations as she started this program, she put it this way: "I've grown more and more uncomfortable with my weight. Every year, a few more pounds have crept onto my body. I know that I'd feel better about myself if I could get rid of the roll of flesh around my waist or fit into the clothes in my closet that I haven't been able to wear for so long. That's my main health goal—to lose the extra weight that I've carried for so long."

Here is Linda's list of Health Goals:

1. Lose 30 pounds.
2. Take three inches off my waistline.
3. Relieve my aches and pains.
4. Sleep better at night.
5. Feel healthier overall!

A man named Ronald told me that while he had achieved more success in the computer business than he ever could have imagined, he had paid a heavy price for it. "I've just turned forty-five," he said, "and I've gained about twenty-five pounds in the past decade. That really upsets me. To make matters worse, I feel completely worn out by the end of the day. I've got new health problems, too—high blood pressure and back pain—that are making me worry. My doctor was pretty clear about it; he said I *had* to start taking better care of myself. No ifs, ands, or buts about it. And he said I'd have to find a way to become more physically active. So here I am. I need some help."

When Ronald began this program, he wrote down the following list of Health Goals, all of which had numbers in them:

1. Lose 25 pounds.
2. Feel 10 years younger.
3. Lower my blood pressure by 20 points.
4. Become twice as energetic as I am today.
5. Live to be 100!

Your own Health Goals should be just that—your own! Don't lose weight to impress others—do it because it would make *you* feel better about yourself and because it's good for your health. Put your needs and desires first for a change. By keeping these goals realistic, you won't be setting yourself up for failure. By making them specific, you'll have a clearer vision of where you're headed and a better chance of getting there. By writing them down below (and on a three-by-five card that you can carry with you), you'll strengthen your commitment to actively pursue them. Refer to these target goals frequently during the next 42 days. Unlike your overall life goals (in Chapter 11), these are specifically targeted at your health. Write them down now:

My Health Goals are:

1. _____

2. _____

3. _____

4. _____

5. _____

Although not everyone finds it necessary to list their Health Goals, many people find this process to be an additional motivation as this program unfolds.

PUTTING IT ALL TOGETHER

Well, are you ready? It's finally time to roll up your sleeves. The many components of *Metabolize* need to be merged into a cohesive success plan. Every element of this program can blend effortlessly into the others, and when that happens, each of them can provide synergistic support for the others. You will be the beneficiary when that happens.

Here are the five key steps to getting *Metabolize* off the ground:

STEP ONE: EATING FOR YOUR TYPE

It is crucial that you follow the diet for your Metabolic Type as closely as possible. That's an absolute! Look at the eating plan for your Type, and you'll see that there are plenty of "allowable" foods. You'll have a lot of freedom and choice within the context of consuming a diet with the optimal nutrient ratios for your Type.

Despite what you've heard in the past about weight-loss plans, it is even more important to support your metabolic individuality than to re-duce the number of calories you consume. By eating the right way, with protein, carbohydrates, and fat in the proper ratio, your metabolism will function at its peak level. Perhaps with other diets you've tried, you were eating too much protein for your own good; on this program, you'll be eating just the proper amount. Or maybe you were consuming too much fat; now you'll be at the right level. And when that happens, your body will function like an automobile that is burning its fuel cleanly, running more smoothly, and lasting longer than less efficient cars. With optimal metabolic functioning, *you'll* last longer, too! You can expect to max out your genetic potential and enjoy greater longevity.

In the short term, as you burn your "fuel" more efficiently, your weight will gradually decline, without the need for becoming obsessed with counting those pesky, annoying calories.

STEP TWO: SUPPLEMENTS

Use supplementation to support your Metabolic Type diet. The best place to start is with a single multivitamin-multimineral tablet each day. When you're shopping for the right product, read labels carefully to ensure that you'll be getting a full range of nutrients. If possible, choose supplements that are part of a food matrix, meaning that the vitamin and mineral molecules are interlaced with protein, carbohydrates, and fat. Look for terms like "food based" or "food matrix" on the label. Refer to Chapter 7 for more information about these supplements. Also, products such as Metabolize™ Nutri-Shake and Nutri-Bar are designed for use in this pro-gram.

STEP THREE: BELLY BREATHING

For most of your life, you probably haven't given much thought to your breathing. But it is really amazing how something that you take for granted can have such a powerful influence on your health. By breathing deeply and rhythmically from the belly, you can fully oxygenate your blood supply, calm your nervous system, and reduce the negative effects of stress in your life. For that reason, you need to make a conscious effort to breathe deep in the belly (diaphragmatic or belly breathing) rather than up in the chest (thoracic or chest breathing).

How can you ensure that proper breathing becomes part of your everyday life? Begin to condition your breathing reflex so that you inhale and exhale properly *all* of the time; in short, you want belly breathing to become a habit that you don't even have to think about. So for at least the first seven days of this program (and longer if you wish), incorporate the following exercises into your life. Altogether, they'll take up less than 20 minutes a day. But don't worry about this time lost: I guarantee that you'll more than make up for those minutes through increased productivity during the rest of the day. Here they are:

✔ Practice belly breathing for five minutes twice a day—just after awakening in the morning, and just before going to bed. This will help spread relaxation throughout your body.
✔ Take three belly breaths before each meal, either right before or just after sitting down at the dining-room table.
✔ Twice during the day, take a short break, sit in a chair, look out the window, and belly breathe for three minutes.

STEP FOUR: THE ENERGY MOVEMENTS

Get moving—but not with just any type of movement. The key here is the Seven No-Sweat Energy Movements. For at least the next 21 (or better yet, 42) days, I recommend doing all of these movements twice a day (it will take only seven to ten minutes to perform them all); after that, once a day is fine, although don't limit yourself if you want to do more.

Unlike most health programs, *Metabolize* doesn't require you to work out until you're worn out. The Energy Movements are smooth and fluid, and you'll begin feeling the benefits right away. As their name suggests, they'll energize you—a natural pick-me-up even when you're feeling dog-tired. They'll extinguish the tension that may leave you frayed and frazzled. Internally, they'll promote efficient oxygen exchange that helps ensure optimal metabolism.

Avoid doing the Energy Movements immediately after eating. Better times are an hour after eating, just before a meal, upon awakening, or prior to going to bed. Expect to feel great almost immediately, with only an occasional side effect. (Some people have short-lived hamstring sore-ness.) If you feel any persistent burning or pinching sensations, however, STOP! This is a sign that the movements have detected a weakness that, to be safe, may need a physician's attention.

STEP FIVE: A NEW ATTITUDE

Your mind can be a powerful weapon in a program like this one. So refor-mulate your thinking, beginning today. Make sure your attitude aids and abets everything you're trying to accomplish.

For example, do you *truly* believe that all of the Health Goals that you listed earlier are achievable? If you have any doubts, you're starting with an anchor tied around your waist. Rather than focusing on the pos-sibility of failure ("This diet probably won't work for me, just like all of the others!"), you need to set aside self-sabotaging thoughts and get an "attitude transplant."

Don't underestimate the power of a positive attitude. Your frame of mind is crucial. Through positive self-talk ("I am getting closer to my goals, meal by meal"), you can help ensure your success with this pro-gram. Instill some positive self-talk into your thinking every day, and no-tice the difference. Refer to Chapter 10 to refresh your memory on how to turn your attitude around.

SLIP SLIDING AWAY

Whether you're 10, 20, 40, or 100 pounds overweight, you probably want to get rid of it all—now! Patience, it seems, is a rare commodity, particu-larly when it comes to weight loss. Many people want to look thinner for a special occasion like an upcoming wedding or a high school reunion.

But if you're looking for pipe-dream promises about instantaneous, overnight weight loss, you haven't found them here. Sorry! *The only way to lose weight fast is to lose it in an unhealthy way.* Nothing could be more counterproductive to the goals of this program.

But don't feel disappointed: You *will* lose your excess weight on *Me-tabolize,* even though it won't all happen with lightning speed. Don't count on losing 42 pounds in 42 days. That requires a starvation diet, and bread and water have never been my style.

So what can you realistically expect? I think it's pretty impressive: Most people using the *Metabolize* program have shed an average of two to three pounds a week. Just by getting their nutrient ratios in order and thus making their metabolism more efficient, they've set themselves on a steady course of weight loss. You might be able to increase your weight loss further by incorporating an active exercise program—perhaps 20 to 30 minutes of walking or jogging three to five times a week—into your routine.

Remember, if you're losing two or three pounds a week, slow and steady wins the race. People who had failed on many other diets finally lost weight for good on this one. The same success can happen to you. So give it a try. If you adopt every element of this program, you won't have to worry about your weight. It will take care of itself.

So be *patient.* (There's that terrible word again!) I know you'll be happy with the results.

"Slow Down, You're Eating Too Fast"

Many (but not all) overweight people eat faster than normal-weight individuals. That's a fact of life. And when they gobble down their food at the speed of the Concorde supersonic jet, they simply get more of it into their stomachs before their brains recognize feelings of satiation and convince them to put down the fork.

Consciously slowing down will help conquer that problem. Most research shows that your brain requires about 20 minutes to realize that you're full. So the rest is pretty simple to understand: If you eat slowly, you'll consume less food by the time this 20-minute period is up.

If weight loss is your goal, I suggest that you try to eat at least 25 percent slower in the first seven days of *Metabolize.* That's right, 25 percent slower! Just the thought of it may make your silverware shudder. But rather than thinking of it as a disruption of the way you eat, reframe it so that it becomes a way to enjoy your food more. Chew slowly. Fully savor the flavor and the texture of your food. Turn eating into a thoroughly hedonistic experience by letting every bite linger in your mouth for several extra seconds. Put your fork down between bites, and concentrate on the food as it bathes your palate. Notice how much you're enjoying it.

"I AM . . ." STATEMENTS

As a final assignment in this chapter, I'd like you to use the space below to reaffirm or reshape the positive Performance Talk that you created in Chapter 10. Remember, these are positive "I am . . ." statements that will support you through the next 21 days times 2 of this program. They are statements such as "I am enjoying belly breathing because it makes me calmer and more self-centered." Or "I am choosing healthy food, meal after meal." Or "I am healthy and love performing the Energy Movements."

In the exercise below, you can use many of the original Performance Talk statements that you've already created. But now, with the entire program in mind, you may decide to formulate some new ones. They should be specific and reinforce the commitment you've made to *Metabolize* and to the renewal of your health. Go ahead and write at least five "I am . . ." statements below:

1. "I am _____."
2. "I am _____."
3. "I am _____."
4. "I am _____."
5. "I am _____."

As you did before, transfer these statements to a three-by-five card. Then carry the card in your pocket or purse during the day, tape it to a mirror, or set it on the dashboard of your car. Refer to it whenever you have a few moments. Say the statements aloud. They can be inspirational and motivational. Even if you don't believe them fully yet, the power of saying them will give your mind a track to follow.

Some people also benefit from rewriting these statements on a new three-by-five card each morning for the next 21 days times 2. Change them if you'd like from what you wrote the day before, or keep them the same. Either way, the act of writing them anew will reinforce your commitment and keep you emotionally strong throughout the next six weeks. Good health is a process, not an event—and this can be an important part of that process.

There are two other steps that I'd like you to take on a weekly basis—that is, on days 7, 14, 21, and so on:

✔ Review your Hierarchy of Values. If appropriate, update them. As you look them over and perhaps fine-tune them, strengthen your resolve to make them the driving forces in your life.

✔ Review the Health Goals that you created earlier in this chapter. If there are moments when you falter in this program—perhaps drifting away from the diet for a few meals, or skipping the Energy Movements for a couple days—glance at your Health Goals again. Visualize yourself living your life as though you had already reached them, whether they're to feel like you're 30 years old instead of 40, or to shed 15 pounds that have stubbornly clung to your body for years. Use these positive images to get you back on track and moving again in the direction of good health.

META-BITE

Review and update your Hierarchy of Values and Health Goals each week. Get excited about your life.

ROGER'S STORY

About a year ago, a businessman named Roger asked for my help in adopting the *Metabolize* program. Although he was very successful (at least financially), he was very unhappy. At age 35, he had little enthusiasm left for his work, and his marriage was disintegrating. He always felt overtired and overspent. Roger knew that there were a lot of things in his life that he needed to change, but he didn't know where or how to begin. I suggested that he start with his health.

"I hate my job," Roger told me. "And I'm not so sure about my wife anymore. But you're right—if anything in my life is going to get any better, my health has to improve."

With my guidance, Roger began eating according to his Metabolic Type. He adjusted his nutrient ratios, adding a little more vegetables, fruits, and protein to his diet and decreasing his fat intake. He also reduced the wheat-based carbohydrates and some of the simple carbohydrates in his diet, which helped minimize his mood swings. At the same time, Roger adopted the other elements of this program: He began breathing and moving the right way, and he shifted his attitude in a more positive direction. "I was a little nervous about the attitude thing," he told me later, with only a bit of sarcasm in his voice. "I was afraid that if I got too positive, I might start liking my job, and I *really* didn't want to do that!"

Within 72 hours, Roger began feeling noticeably better. "There was a fog that kind of lifted from my head," he told me. For the first time in years, he felt energized from morning until night. His attitude changed, and yes, as it did, he started to enjoy his job more. With this new and improved outlook on life, his marriage began to get better, too.

As Roger progressed through *Metabolize,* from the first 21-day cycle to the second, he said that the program was becoming easier for him to follow, week by week. After a while, it just became part of him. He no longer had to give it the careful thought that he did in the beginning. By the time the program had ended, he had lost 16 pounds without any great effort. "Ken," he told me, "it's not as simple as ABC, but it's pretty close. I wish I had known years ago that changing my diet would make such a difference in how I feel and how I look."

Perhaps most significantly, with the help of his Hierarchy of Values, Roger decided what he really wanted in life, and it included his wife. With a clear head, he recognized that his spouse was still "the girl of my dreams." He embraced his renewed life and saw a new beginning ahead of him. "This program was like having riches buried in my own backyard. It was right there for the taking, but I never knew it until now."

Over the years, I've collected hundreds of case studies like Roger's, showing that this program really works. My own clients have included men and women from all walks of life. All of them had their own goals—from losing weight to regaining their energy and good health. In every case, after identifying their Metabolic Type and honoring and supporting their biochemical individuality, they adopted a health-enhancement program individualized for them. *Metabolize* helped them feel better, sleep sounder, and enjoy a more energetic lifestyle. Even when their primary focus was on losing weight, a lot of other good things happened that promoted their overall good health.

You have a lot of potential inside of you, just bursting to get out. I know this even though we've never met. If you live this program every day, you can release the power within. When you do, you'll discover the simple pleasures of a belt that fits around your waist a little looser than it once did, a bathroom scale that's much more friendly and to your liking, and a mirror that tells you it's okay to remove your clothes! No matter what your age, *Metabolize* really can produce some quite magnificent results. No matter what your health status is today, you can begin to transform your life for the better.

HOW ARE YOU DOING?

Use the logs below to keep track of your progress in *Metabolize*. Although you should also use the charts at the end of Chapter 5 to monitor the food you eat, the tables below will give you a broader overview of how you're doing with the entire program. By keeping this ongoing record, you can see clearly what you're doing right, as well as the areas where you need to improve.

There are enough logs here to track your progress for the first week of the program. (I suggest you photocopy the charts so you have enough for the following two weeks as well.) Throughout each day (or at the end of the day if it's more convenient), check the appropriate boxes for the activities that you've completed. Then, when looking back at how you've done, scan for those areas without checkmarks and where you need to do better. Note these problems or weaknesses and then make a special effort to improve, starting the following morning.

DAY 1

Date: _____

Eating for Your Metabolic Type
I ate in the proper nutrient ratios for:
- ☐ Breakfast
- ☐ Lunch
- ☐ Dinner
- ☐ Snack 1
- ☐ Snack 2

Supplementation
- ☐ I took a multivitamin/multimineral tablet today.

Breathing
I practiced belly breathing for five minutes twice today:
- ☐ Upon awakening in the morning
- ☐ Just before bedtime at night

I took three belly breaths just before each meal:
- ☐ Breakfast
- ☐ Lunch
- ☐ Dinner

I performed belly breathing for three minutes, 2 times today, while thinking of a relaxing place:
- ☐ Practice session 1
- ☐ Practice session 2

Seven No-Sweat Energy Movements
I performed the seven energy movements twice today:
- ☐ Morning session
- ☐ Evening session

Attitude
- ☐ I used self-talk to maintain a positive attitude for this program.
- ☐ I saw myself as a success today.

Day 2

Date: _____

Eating for Your Metabolic Type

I ate in the proper nutrient ratios for:

- ☐ Breakfast
- ☐ Lunch
- ☐ Dinner
- ☐ Snack 1
- ☐ Snack 2

Supplementation

- ☐ I took a multivitamin-multimineral tablet today.

Breathing

I practiced belly breathing for five minutes twice today:

- ☐ Upon awakening in the morning
- ☐ Just before bedtime at night

I took three belly breaths just before each meal:

- ☐ Breakfast
- ☐ Lunch
- ☐ Dinner

I performed belly breathing for three minutes, 2 times today, while thinking of a relaxing place:

- ☐ Practice session 1
- ☐ Practice session 2

Seven No-Sweat Energy Movements

I performed the seven energy movements twice today:

- ☐ Morning session
- ☐ Evening session

Attitude

- ☐ I used "self-talk" to maintain a positive attitude for this program.
- ☐ I saw myself as a success today.

DAY 3

Date: _____

EATING FOR YOUR METABOLIC TYPE

I ate in the proper nutrient ratios for:

- ☐ Breakfast
- ☐ Lunch
- ☐ Dinner
- ☐ Snack 1
- ☐ Snack 2

SUPPLEMENTATION

☐ I took a multivitamin-multimineral tablet today.

BREATHING

I practiced belly breathing for five minutes twice today:

- ☐ Upon awakening in the morning
- ☐ Just before bedtime at night

I took three belly breaths just before each meal:

- ☐ Breakfast
- ☐ Lunch
- ☐ Dinner

I performed belly breathing for three minutes, 2 times today, while thinking of a relaxing place:

- ☐ Practice session 1
- ☐ Practice session 2

SEVEN NO-SWEAT ENERGY MOVEMENTS

I performed the seven energy movements twice today:

- ☐ Morning session
- ☐ Evening session

ATTITUDE

- ☐ I used self-talk to maintain a positive attitude for this program.
- ☐ I saw myself as a success today.

DAY 4

Date: _____

EATING FOR YOUR METABOLIC TYPE

I ate in the proper nutrient ratios for:

- ☐ Breakfast
- ☐ Lunch
- ☐ Dinner
- ☐ Snack 1
- ☐ Snack 2

SUPPLEMENTATION

☐ I took a multivitamin/multimineral tablet today.

BREATHING

I practiced belly breathing for five minutes twice today:

- ☐ Upon awakening in the morning
- ☐ Just before bedtime at night

I took three belly breaths just before each meal:

- ☐ Breakfast
- ☐ Lunch
- ☐ Dinner

I performed belly breathing for three minutes, 2 times today, while thinking of a relaxing place:

- ☐ Practice session 1
- ☐ Practice session 2

SEVEN NO-SWEAT ENERGY MOVEMENTS

I performed the seven energy movements twice today:

- ☐ Morning session
- ☐ Evening session

ATTITUDE

☐ I used self-talk to maintain a positive attitude for this program.

DAY 5

Date: _____

EATING FOR YOUR METABOLIC TYPE
I ate in the proper nutrient ratios for:
- ☐ Breakfast
- ☐ Lunch
- ☐ Dinner
- ☐ Snack 1
- ☐ Snack 2

SUPPLEMENTATION
- ☐ I took a multivitamin-multimineral tablet today.

BREATHING
I practiced belly breathing for five minutes twice today:
- ☐ Upon awakening in the morning
- ☐ Just before bedtime at night

I took three belly breaths just before each meal:
- ☐ Breakfast
- ☐ Lunch
- ☐ Dinner

I performed belly breathing for three minutes, 2 times today, while thinking of a relaxing place:
- ☐ Practice session 1
- ☐ Practice session 2

SEVEN NO-SWEAT ENERGY MOVEMENTS
I performed the seven energy movements twice today:
- ☐ Morning session
- ☐ Evening session

ATTITUDE
- ☐ I used self-talk to maintain a positive attitude for this program.
- ☐ I saw myself as a success today.

DAY 6

Date: _____

EATING FOR YOUR METABOLIC TYPE

I ate in the proper nutrient ratios for:

- ☐ Breakfast
- ☐ Lunch
- ☐ Dinner
- ☐ Snack 1
- ☐ Snack 2

SUPPLEMENTATION

☐ I took a multivitamin-multimineral tablet today.

BREATHING

I practiced belly breathing for five minutes twice today:

- ☐ Upon awakening in the morning
- ☐ Just before bedtime at night

I took three belly breaths just before each meal:

- ☐ Breakfast
- ☐ Lunch
- ☐ Dinner

I performed belly breathing for three minutes, 2 times today, while thinking of a relaxing place:

- ☐ Practice session 1
- ☐ Practice session 2

SEVEN NO-SWEAT ENERGY MOVEMENTS

I performed the seven energy movements twice today:

- ☐ Morning session
- ☐ Evening session

ATTITUDE

- ☐ I used self-talk to maintain a positive attitude for this program.
- ☐ I saw myself as a success today.

DAY 7

Date: _____

EATING FOR YOUR METABOLIC TYPE
I ate in the proper nutrient ratios for:
- ☐ Breakfast
- ☐ Lunch
- ☐ Dinner
- ☐ Snack 1
- ☐ Snack 2

SUPPLEMENTATION
- ☐ I took a multivitamin-multimineral tablet today.

BREATHING
I practiced belly breathing for five minutes twice today:
- ☐ Upon awakening in the morning
- ☐ Just before bedtime at night

I took three belly breaths just before each meal:
- ☐ Breakfast
- ☐ Lunch
- ☐ Dinner

I performed belly breathing for three minutes, 2 times today, while thinking of a relaxing place:
- ☐ Practice session 1
- ☐ Practice session 2

SEVEN NO-SWEAT ENERGY MOVEMENTS
I performed the seven energy movements twice a day:
- ☐ Morning session
- ☐ Evening session

ATTITUDE
- ☐ I used self-talk to maintain a positive attitude for this program.
- ☐ I saw myself as a success today.

The 21-Day Action Plan times 2 gives you all the tools you need to reach your goals and improve your life. So get started. Stick with it. Enjoy the changes you'll begin to experience.

14

Fine-Tuning Metabolize

> *"Never eat more than you can lift!"*
> —MISS PIGGY

By now, you've certainly gotten the message that one diet isn't right for everyone. As you've learned, the diet that's ideal for you may not be good for me—or even for your own family members. If you've failed on diets in the past, it's because you needed a customized program that recognizes your own unique metabolic individuality. And because that never happened until now, no wonder you may have a long history of one failed diet after another.

I hope your experience is finally different this time. You have probably already enjoyed some success—and will continue to have even more of it—because this program is not lying to your metabolism. People are not the same biochemically. Their paths to good health are not the same.

Remember, this program is not about transforming you into the next Cindy Crawford or Mel Gibson. It's about looking and feeling the best that you possibly can. It's about being healthy in the skin that you're already in. It's about living the longest and healthiest life that your genetics will allow. It's about finally putting behind you the way you may have always dieted in the past—skipping meals, starving yourself, gulping diet drinks, dashing off to weight-loss clinics and "fat farms," and popping the latest generation of diet pills. Thankfully, those days are gone.

Whether your initial hope was to lose five pounds or 50 pounds, or simply to feel better, this program is the optimal approach to help you reach your goals. As the days and weeks pass and as you move from the first 21-day cycle through the second 21 days, continue to conscientiously follow the program and monitor your progress. Resolve to do as well or better in each succeeding week. Keep track of your strengths and weaknesses. What are you doing well? And what areas do you still need to work on? Also, do you feel more energetic? And are you managing stress better?

> **META-BITE**
>
> **R**esolve to do better with Metabolize *each week than you did the week before. Enjoy the process.*

FINE-TUNING THE PROCESS

Life is beautiful. But like life itself, every weight-control and health-enhancement program may present a pothole or two on the road to success. Just when you're making both short- and long-term progress with *Metabolize,* and wondering how life could really be this good, an unexpected lapse may raise its unwelcome head—and splat! You might give in to a craving for a "taboo" food—and then find yourself bingeing for days. You may regain a pound or two—or more.

Slips and backsliding happen to everyone. Simply be prepared to fight back. You may have some troubleshooting to do along the way, and the problem areas are not always obvious. At times, any fine-tuning needs to be quite subtle.

For example, let's say that your primary goal has been to lose 20 pounds. And although you seem to be following every element of the program, the scale isn't cooperating. At best you're shedding a pound a week, and some weeks nothing at all. What's wrong?

You need to reevaluate whether you're actually eating according to the optimal nutrient ratio for your Metabolic Type. Is your ratio of protein, carbohydrates, and fat really on target? If it is, are you choosing foods from your approved list, or are you frequently straying from it? If everything seems in order, take a bow—and then consider making modest reductions in the amount of calories you consume—from 1,800 to 1,600 calories, for example. Slightly decrease the number of calories you're eating, while still keeping your ratios in alignment with your Metabolic Type. By eating in sync with your proper ratio, your metabolism will continue to function efficiently, which should keep you pointed in the direction of weight loss. But if those extra pounds are stubbornly clinging to your frame, then cutting calories very modestly makes sense—although you should *not* overdo it. Trim your calories by just 100 to 200 calories a day, and see what happens.

Another common problem area is feeling hungry within two hours of eating. You may have breakfast at home at 7:30, and by 9:30, you're ready to grab the doughnuts from every nearby desk at work. If that sounds familiar, take a close look at your diet. Again, perhaps your nutrient ratios and your food choices aren't quite on target. If they're not right, that's probably what's drawing you like a magnet to the refrigerator just an hour or two after your last meal.

But what if you really are being true to your ratios and are still having difficulties? Here is what I suggest:

✔ If you're hungry two hours after eating, try making some adjustments to your diet. Even minor shifts in the amounts of each nutrient group can often make a big difference in finding a ratio that fully supports your biochemical individuality. For most people, the best formula is to slightly increase the protein and fat in the diet, while decreasing the carbohydrates a little. Try it and see how you feel. A little tweaking like this may be all you need.

✔ If these adjustments don't seem to be the answer—for example, if you eat lunch at noon and are absolutely starving by the 2:30 coffee break, then shift into the next troubleshooting strategy: Add an additional small meal at midafternoon, fitting it in between lunch and dinner. As I pointed out in Chapter 6, people who experience between-meal hunger are probably fast oxidizers of their food. To address the problem, get some food into your stomach before those hunger pangs start growling, using your nutrient ratios as a guide to your food choices. The same is true for midmorning; if you're hungry a couple hours after breakfast, add a small meal or snack between breakfast and lunch.

Remember, there is nothing sacred about eating breakfast at 7 A.M., lunch at noon and dinner at 6 P.M. Your body simply may not function optimally when you go five or six hours between meals. You may need to add an additional meal or two during the day, and/or adjust the times of your three main meals. Once you find an eating pattern that works for you, try to stick with it consistently, day after day.

✓ Keep the following caveat in mind when you're adding an extra meal or two to your day—eating four or five (or occasionally even six) times a day instead of three: Avoid boosting your caloric intake by modestly decreasing the amount of calories you eat in your other meals. Believe me, five or six regular-sized meals a day aren't the key to success in weight loss! But if you're snacking by design and planning those snacks so they support your nutrient ratios, they can be an important tool for reaching your weight-loss goals. For the most part, avoid snack foods; if you're looking for something that can be eaten quickly, select a nutritious food bar (like the Bioblend Metabolize bar mentioned in Appendix B); if you read the labels, you'll find some that closely coincide with your own fat-protein-carbohydrate ratio.

✓ If the pounds just aren't coming off, try eliminating wheat from your diet. Many people have an allergic reaction to wheat, characterized by symptoms like fatigue and mouth sores, and disruptions in their metabolism that make losing weight difficult. Take the wheat out of your meals for a couple weeks, and see if it makes a difference.

✓ When you're not thinking as clearly as you'd like, you may need to slightly increase the percentage of carbohydrates in your diet, while reducing your protein and fat intake a small amount. Carbohydrates are a primary source of glucose—which is brain food—and even a very modest rise in carbos can make a noticeable difference in your thought processes.

✓ Now, what if you seem to be doing everything right, but everything seems to be going wrong? Your weight's up and your energy's down! Help! Well, when you're not reaching your goals on this program, here's another important thing to consider: Medications may be creating havoc with your internal biochemistry. Are you taking thyroid medication, for example, which can put the brakes on a normal metabolic rate? Or is the normal functioning of your body being sabotaged by a chronic illness or the drugs you're taking for it? Talk to your doctor about the medications you're taking; if they could be the saboteur within, maybe you can switch to another drug with fewer disruptive side effects.

By the way, in some cases, allergies or chemical exposure could be responsible for your inability to reach your goals with this program. Talk to your doctor about undergoing tests to determine whether allergies or another environmental problem could be sabotaging your good health. You could be sensitive to common allergenic foods (corn, wheat, peanuts, eggs, strawberries, fish, many additives and preservatives), and eliminating them from your diet could get you back on track. Contact the Biodynamics Institute for more information about these health concerns.

Even if you haven't lost weight as rapidly as you had hoped, don't wave the white flag quite yet. Keep in mind that muscle tissue is denser than fat, so as you rebuild a little muscle (thanks to the Seven No-Sweat Energy Movements), you might actually lose weight a bit more slowly than if you were following an extremely low-calorie fad diet that caused muscle destruction. Enjoy the fact that your body is becoming firmer and stronger. Perhaps get a little more physical activity. If you're persistent, you *will* succeed with this program, even if you're losing weight at a rate slower than two to three pounds a week. Although most people will begin to notice changes after the first 48 hours on this program, it may take you the full 42 days to get your metabolism fully in balance and to enjoy the physical goals that you're trying to reach. Be patient. Once your metabolism is in balance, the pounds will come off quicker.

Also, let me make this point very clear: *Do not let the bathroom scale be your only measure of success.* As you've seen, this is a multifaceted program designed to improve your overall health, not just your body weight. So if you feel better—perhaps enjoying more energy during the day and sleeping more soundly at night, noticing improvements in your muscle tone and decreases in your blood pressure—*Metabolize* has been a sensational plan for you. The scale reflects only your body weight; it's not a gauge of the other aspects of good health. And while many people look only at their weight as the barometer of success, expand your horizons a little. You're probably doing better than you think.

SHAKING UP YOUR METABOLISM

There is one more important strategy to consider. It is primarily for people who still have more weight to lose after 42 days of this program. At this point, your metabolism may have adapted to a 1,600- to 1,800-calorie diet, and it's time to "shake things up" and get you off the plateau on which you may find yourself. It's time for a metabolic makeover!

This strategy involves very briefly eating *more* calories, then reducing your caloric intake, and then raising it again. It's a way of jarring your metabolic rate out of a slowdown or an "I'm starving" mode that makes further weight loss very difficult. Unless you do something to change it, you might have trouble losing more weight.

Here's how this technique works (it is sometimes called "Up, Down & Under"):

✔ For one to two days, *increase* your total food intake by 200 to 500 calories per day. Keep your ratio the same, but add one or two snacks, or increase your portion sizes in your meals. This modest increase in calories will move your metabolism out of its comfort zone, albeit briefly.

✔ Next, for the following five to six days, return to your baseline caloric intake—1,600 or 1,800 calories a day. However, there is one exception during this period: Choose a day in the middle of this five to six days, and eat *fewer* calories than you've been doing by about 200 to 500 a day—thus decreasing your consumption to perhaps 1,300 calories if you've been on the 1,600-calorie plan. But remember, this is only for one day. You can achieve this lower level by cutting out a snack or two, emphasizing more fruits and vegetables in your diet, or leaving food on your plate while still maintaining your proper ratio.

✔ Then, repeat this cycle at least one more time—first increasing your caloric intake, followed by a return to baseline (with one day of decreased calories in the middle).

✔ Finally, return to the regular program, eating at your normal 1,600- or 1,800-calorie level for the long term.

Get the picture? This process will jar your metabolism out of any rut it has fallen into. So don't panic if you feel stuck and try slashing your caloric intake drastically for an extended time period; this will only get you into more trouble, including eventual binges. Instead, use the technique described above to shake up your metabolism and get it back on track so that it works as efficiently as it did in the earliest days of this program. It will conquer plateaus and keep you from feeling frustrated.

WHEN YOU GET OFF TRACK . . .

Although we've talked about lapses before, they're worth reemphasizing as you look to your future with *Metabolize*. What happens, for example, when dietary diversions occur unintentionally, with almost unconscious lapses into poor eating choices that seem to be undermining all the progress you've made? Or what if you've skipped doing the No-Sweat Energy Movements and just keep letting one missed workout session pile on top of another?

Don't panic, and don't give up! As you read in Chapter 10, *everyone* has a lapse now and then. An occasional lapse isn't that big a deal. (One dictionary defines *lapse* as "a slight error typically due to forgetfulness or inattention"—I think you can deal with a *slight* error, don't you?) So stop beating up on yourself. Keep in mind that *Metabolize* isn't a restrictive program; it's a system for moving in the direction of maximizing your metabolism at the cellular level. If you make a "mistake," don't assume that all is lost—because it isn't. This isn't a failure, it's feedback.

Don't let disappointment, frustration, or feelings of failure throw you off course. Once you've refocused your attention and your energy where they belong, conduct a little self-evaluation on why your lapse may have occurred. Were you overwhelmed with deadlines at work? Or did you just have a big argument with your spouse, and you overate to soothe your stress? Did a series of Christmas and New Year's parties take you prisoner and overwhelm you with irresistible dietary temptations? Or was your father seriously ill in the hospital, and the last thing on your mind was conscientious meal-planning? If you can identify the spoiler, be especially wary of it in the future. Consider the slip to be a worthwhile learning experience.

The big risk, according to Dr. Kelly Brownell of the Yale Center for Eating and Weight Disorders, is when "lapse becomes relapse and then collapse." But the good news is that as this program becomes a part of you, slips will become much less common. For some extra support, consider using a Metabolize™ coach (see the Appendix for contact information for the Biodynamics Institute).

"CAN MY METABOLIC TYPE CHANGE?"

You were born with a particular Metabolic Type. You can thank your genetics for that. But amazingly, your Type can change over time. As I noted in Chapter 3, a number of factors, from sickness to stress to pollutants, can alter your Type at any point in life, including while you're on this 42-day program. The functioning of some of your organs—from the liver to the pancreas—can change, often simply due to aging, and this can alter your Type.

Meta-Check

What if you find yourself having difficulty losing weight? What can you do to shed those extra pounds? In addition to the strategies discussed in this chapter, here are some other things to try:

➔ Check to make sure you are eating primarily from your Preferred list.

➔ Monitor your ratios—they matter!

➔ Do the Seven No-Sweat Energy Movements three times a day.

➔ If your Metabolic Type is Lean or Super-Lean, incorporate strength training to your program (see page 208); if you are Mixed, focus on modest aerobic exercise (page 204) and modest strength training; if you are Clean or Super-Clean, increase your aerobic exercise even further.

➔ Reduce your caloric intake by one snack or by a total of 200 calories.

Occasionally, I've worked with clients who had plenty of success on *Metabolize*, losing weight and reaching their other Health Goals. But then something unexpected happened. After months or even a year or two of maintaining their improvements, a tidal wave of problems smacked them where it hurts. They gained a few pounds—and sometimes more than a few. They felt run-down and always in need of a nap. And all of this happened even though they still conscientiously ate the diet for their Type.

I've encouraged these people to take the Metabolic Type self-test again. When they have, most have found that their Type had changed. Super-Cleans became Cleans, while Mixeds and Leans shifted as well. With that information in hand, they altered their diet, began eating in sync with a new nutrient ratio—and started losing weight and regained their energy. Voilà!

If you notice unexpected negative changes in your overall health, including your body weight, retake the self-test in Chapter 4. You may find that you are no longer the Type you once were. If that's the case, turn to Chapter 5, and shift to the diet appropriate for your new Type.

WHAT ABOUT THE FUTURE?

Once you've completed the 42-day program, there is more on your agenda. Do you really want to go back to eating the old way? Do you really want to return to a sedentary life and relegate the Seven Energy Movements to a distant memory? Not if you want the improvements in your health to continue.

I'd like you to consider the 42 days of this program just the beginning. As you look ahead and contemplate sticking with *Metabolize* for the long term, keep in mind that you won't have to be as rigid as you were in the first six weeks. But you can't retreat to your old habits, either. As you move forward, keep your nutrient ratios at or very close to where they've been for the previous six weeks. At the same time, if you occasionally stray by eating a food not on the recommended list for your Type, it won't be the end of the world. But notice how you feel, and ask yourself if it was worth it.

After completing the entire 42-day cycle, you should be feeling a surge of good health and balance throughout your body. When that happens, you *can* finally begin to consume some of the foods that weren't on the eating list for your Type, in a so-called "42-day test." While continuing to eat for your Type most of the time and for the foreseeable future, you *can* now splurge once in a while by eating a food that you love but that isn't on your recommended list. After the first six weeks of *Metabolize*, you can periodically try these "taboo" foods and see how your body reacts to them. Most people won't even notice any effect of having taken this nutritional detour. Others, however, may actually feel a little out of sync physically or mentally, and it may take a day or two for their body to rebound. Whatever the case, let this occasional "cheating" occur by design and by having a treat now and then, rather than by succumbing to temptation unexpectedly and then overdoing it.

In fact, here's my bottom-line recommendation: After 42 days, you can gradually begin to reintroduce "off limits" foods into your diet, one at a time, and see how you react to them. First of all, you'll find that if you indulge those cravings once in a while, it can help prevent feelings of deprivation ("I've *got* to eat a candy bar!!!") that can lead to uncontrollable bingeing. So don't feel any guilt. Just enjoy that "taboo" food without losing control.

But also keep the following in mind: Some bodies don't digest certain foods very well. Or they're prone to having allergic reactions to particular foods, or a rush of insulin will be released by the pancreas, creating all kinds of cravings. The idea, then, is to stay away from those foods for 42 days; then, at a point where your body is finally in balance, if you want to try to introduce them and see how your body adjusts, that's fine. Approach these foods cautiously, and listen to your body for feedback on whether you can start eating them with regularity. But if you develop any of the following symptoms, that's a message that this food isn't supportive of your good health, and that you may even be allergic to it:

- ✔ headaches
- ✔ flatulence
- ✔ itchy eyes
- ✔ stuffy nose
- ✔ sore throat
- ✔ swollen glands

✔ canker sores
✔ coughing or wheezing
✔ heartburn
✔ joint stiffness
✔ hives or skin rashes

When symptoms like these develop and particularly if they persist, I'd advise staying away from the problematic foods altogether or at least significantly minimizing your exposure to them. If you develop indigestion, feel irritable or tired, or awaken with puffy eyes the next morning, for example, these reactions indicate that you should keep your distance for good. On the other hand, if you don't sense any kind of physiological response at all, welcome the food back into your life on occasion.

Remember, even after 42 days, try to stick with your ratios and your list of approved foods as closely as possible. These foods should become the core items in your diet for the rest of your life (unless your Metabolic Type changes). But if you have one or more favorite foods that you've had to avoid for the previous six weeks, conduct your own scientific experiment and see if it can be reintroduced problem-free.

By the way, there really is no bad food. Even foods that don't fit in with your Metabolic Type provide some nutrients; eating a quarter-pound burger with cheese and fries, or an entire extra large pepperoni pizza, is better than starving. If push came to shove, you could survive on that diet (at least until your coronary arteries became hopelessly clogged or an allergic reaction got the best of you). Yet even though there's no *bad* food, there are *better* choices for better health, no matter what your Metabolic Type.

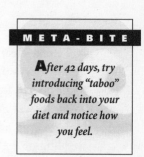

META-BITE

After 42 days, try introducing "taboo" foods back into your diet and notice how you feel.

ONCE YOU REACH YOUR GOALS

When you lose all the weight you want to lose—whether it takes 21 days, 42 days, or longer—you have every reason to feel proud of what you've accomplished. You've persevered and are enjoying the payoff.

As I've suggested, I'd like you to stick with the program at this point.

Of course, weight loss is no longer your primary goal, but good health is. And *Metabolize* can help you maximize your overall health in the months and years ahead.

With weight loss no longer an objective, you can now make some adjustments in what you eat. Although you should continue to prepare meals according to the ratios for your Metabolic Type, you can now consume portions that are a little larger since you're not trying to eat fewer calories than you burn anymore. Try adding 200 calories a day to your meals by increasing portion sizes a little. That may be enough for you to maintain your weight right where you want it. Some people find that they can increase their caloric intake even further without adding to their weight.

As the weeks unfold, reward yourself from time to time for the progress you've made. That reward can be a favorite food, but it doesn't have to be. Take yourself on a shopping spree (perhaps buying clothes that reflect your new, smaller size). Slip into a hot, soothing bath with candles burning nearby. Buy yourself a bouquet of your favorite flowers. Get a massage. Retreat to your favorite weekend vacation spot. You've earned the right to indulge yourself.

SOME FINAL THOUGHTS . . .

As I stressed earlier in the book, there are all kinds of reasons that people decide they want to lose weight and turn their life around for the better. Some people, for example, have asked for my help because they're desperate to lose 25 pounds before a family wedding. Or maybe they want to look great in a bathing suit on a long-awaited trip to Hawaii. Once the wedding or the vacation has come and gone, they tell themselves, "Mission accomplished!" and go back to their old ways—and their old weight.

If you're tempted to do the same, take a moment to reflect on all the progress you've made. Do you really want to let go of that? I'm proud of the accomplishments you've made, and I encourage you to continue unleashing the inner strength that you've shown. There's plenty of truth to the old cliché "When you have your health, you have everything!" And most people can recapture all the good health they want.

So I encourage you to keep going, and to enjoy every step of the journey. You really can have fun along the way as you continue to pursue an optimal level of health and well-being. No matter what your chronological age, you can live at a much lower functional age—that is, you can be a 40-year-old who functions in life as though you were 30; or a 50-year-old who is so healthy that you're able to lead your life as if you were 40. Sure, genetics are important, but so are the decisions you make in life that affect your well-being. You have tremendous potential just bursting to get out and guide you toward achieving a slimmer and healthier body.

If no one else is saying it, let me congratulate you. Be proud of yourself. Feel wonderful about all that you've accomplished so far. You really do feel better, don't you? You really do look more attractive and sexier, don't you?

You're finally taking care of yourself the way you should. You are a real success and have proven what you can achieve when you set your mind to it. You also need to recognize the compelling future that awaits you, if you're willing to make the most of it.

Finally, give the following question some thought:

How often do you have the chance to improve your health?

The answer is: "Every time you take a bite . . . every time you put your body in motion . . . every time your attitude is positive and optimistic . . . and every time you take a breath."

It really is that simple.

Ain't life grand!

Appendix A
Are You Really Overweight?

In 1998, the National Institutes of Health announced new obesity guidelines. Created by a panel of 24 obesity authorities, they concluded that you're "overweight" if you have a body mass index (BMI) of 25 or more (and you're categorized as "obese" with a BMI of 30 or greater).

What is the BMI? It is a correlation between a person's body weight and height. When the panel reached its BMI guidelines, it took into account the research showing that when BMI levels increase to a range of 25 to 29.9 and higher, total cholesterol levels and blood pressure readings also tend to rise, while "good" (HDL) cholesterol levels decrease. And when weight rises to "obese" levels, individuals have a greater likelihood of developing heart disease, strokes, diabetes, and cancer.

To figure out your own BMI, follow these steps:

✔ Take your weight, and multiply it by 0.45. So if the bathroom scale shows 160 pounds, for instance, you'd multiply 160 by 0.45. The answer: 72.

✔ Next, multiply your height (in inches) by 0.025. So if you're five foot six (or 66 inches), multiply 66 by 0.025. The answer is 1.65

✔ Then take the answer in step 2, and multiply it by itself (or square it). In our example, multiply by 1.65. The answer: 2.72.

✔ Finally, take the answer in the first step (72 in our example), and divide it by the answer in the third step (2.72). Thus, 72 divided by 2.72 equals 26.47.

In this example, the individual is overweight, according to government guidelines, with a BMI greater than 25.

Appendix B
Where to Find the Foods in Metabolize

Some of the foods that are incorporated into this program may be unfamiliar to you. Even so, they are probably readily available in stores in your community. Whether you're looking for sprouted wheat bread, adzuki beans, Soyrizo, or Soy Dream, you'll find them in many major supermarkets. In some cases, you might have to go to a specialty market or a health food store. But if you scan the shelves of stores in your city, you'll find everything you need. If you don't see what you want, ask the store manager. (Many stores keep sprouted wheat bread, for example, in the refrigerator or freezer section.)

For information about the Metabolize™ Bioblend products (supplements, drinks, food bars) mentioned in the book, or for additional information about the *Metabolize* program itself, contact the Biodynamics Institute at this address and phone number:

Biodynamics Institute
P.O. Box 1269
San Juan Capistrano, CA 92693
toll-free: 1-800-828-3343
website: *www.metabolize.net*

Appendix C
Create Your Own Metabolize Food Plan

Some people may decide that the sample menus in Chapter 6 aren't quite right for them. Perhaps 1,600 or 1,800 calories a day isn't enough because of their body size. Or perhaps they're a competitive athlete who needs to be consuming more food. The tables below will help you come up with your own formulas to guide you in creating your own unique *Metabolize* diet, while still being true to the ratios for your Metabolic Type. It will help you determine how many calories and grams of protein, fat, and carbohydrate you should be eating for your Type.

1. To determine your intake of calories and grams of *protein:*

   - Multiply your total daily calories by your protein ratio. If you've decided to raise your caloric intake to 2,000, for example, and you are Lean (20% protein), you would do the following:

     2,000 x .20 = 400 total protein calories

Then, to determine the grams of protein you should be aiming for, divide the total protein calories (400 in this example) by 4 calories per gram:

400 divided by 4 = 100 total protein grams.

2. To determine your intake of calories and grams of carbohydrates:

- Multiply your total daily calories by your carbohydrate ratio. If you've decided to raise your caloric intake to 2,000, and you are Lean (60% carbohydrate), you would do the following:

2,000 x .60 = 1200 total carbohydrate calories

Then, to determine the grams of carbohydrates you should be aiming for, divide the total carbohydrate calories (1200 in this example) by 4 calories per gram:

1,200 divided by 4 = 300 total carbohydrate grams

3. To determine your intake of calories and grams of *fat:*

- Multiply your total daily calories by your fat ratio. If you've decided to raise your caloric intake to 2,000, and you are Lean (20% fat), you would do the following:

2,000 x .20 = 400 fat calories

Then, to determined the grams of fat you should be aiming for, divide the total fat calories (400 in this example) by 9 calories per gram:

400 divided by 9 = 44.4 total fat grams

Appendix D
Maximize Your Metabolize Program

The following publications and products from Kenneth Baum can help enhance the program in this book:

✔ *The Seven No-Sweat Energy Movements*
video, 30 minutes
Metabolize Fitness Products

✔ *Metabolize Stretch & Flex*
a "gym in a pocket": strength and flexibility apparatus and instructional video
Metabolize Fitness Products

✔ *The Mental Edge: Maximize Your Sports Potential with the Mind-Body Connection*
a book by Kenneth Baum with Richard Trubo
Perigee Books

✔ *The Mental Edge Training System*
6 audiotapes, video, workbook
The Biodynamics Institute

✔ *The Performance Zone: A Personalized Plan for Increasing Health, Energy and Longevity*
6 audiotapes, workbook
Nightingale-Conant

✔ All of the mental training exercises in *Metabolize* are available on audiotape from the Biodynamics Institute.

For information about these products, contact the Biodynamics Institute at:

1-800-828-3343
website: *www.metabolize.net*

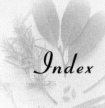

Index

Page numbers in *italics* refer to illustrations.

About Ken Baum's Biodynamics Institute

The Biodynamics Institute has brought together some of the finest researchers in the health and peak performance fields—physicians, psychologists, nutritionists, chiropractors, pharmacists, physical therapists, certified strength and conditioning coaches, and certified personal trainers. All of these experts are dedicated to improving the human condition and unleashing the full potential of every individual.

The Institute was founded by Ken Baum to find real answers to facilitate weight management, optimal health, and peak performance. By drawing upon the expertise of authorities in many fields, the Institute has been able to cut through the maze of theory and research to develop usable, hands-on programs.

As President of the Biodynamics Institute, Ken oversees and provides direction to all of the organization's efforts. He is available as a consultant to individuals, companies, and athletic teams. He is a highly regarded motivational and keynote speaker. Other services from the Biodynamics Institute include:

✔ Personal coaching for the *Metabolize* program
✔ Customized fitness programs developed by the Biodynamics staff
✔ Workshops, seminars and multi-day retreats
✔ Corporate wellness programs
✔ The Biodynamics Newsletter

Contact the Biodynamics Institute by phone: (877) KEN-BAUM

website: *www.metabolize.net*